HEALTH CARE HANDBOOK

A Clear and Concise Guide to the
United States Health Care System

THIRD EDITION

THE
HEALTH CARE
HANDBOOK

A Clear and Concise Guide to the United States Health Care System

THIRD EDITION

Elisabeth Askin, MD

Associate Clinical Professor, Medicine
Department of Medicine
University of California-San Francisco
San Francisco, California

Nathan Moore, MD

Medical Director
BJC Accountable Care Organization
Instructor, Clinical Medicine
Washington University in St. Louis
St. Louis, Missouri

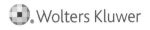. Wolters Kluwer

Philadelphia • Baltimore • New York • London
Buenos Aires • Hong Kong • Sydney • Tokyo

Acquisitions Editor: Joe Cho
Development Editors: Anne Malcolm and Maria McAvey
Editorial Coordinator: Venugopal Loganathan
Marketing Manager: Kirsten Watrud
Production Project Manager: Matt West
Design Manager: Stephen Druding
Manufacturing Coordinator: Beth Welsh
Prepress Vendor: S4Carlisle Publishing Services

Third Edition

9 8 7 6 5 4 3 2 1

Printed in Mexico

Library of Congress Cataloging-in-Publication Data

ISBN-13: 978-1-975200-02-2

Cataloging-in-publication data available on request from the Publisher.

shop.lww.com

QUADM0123

Foreword

Several years ago, I gave a talk on health policy to a group of medical students at my institution. Given that I spend much of my day with practicing physicians who have no hesitation complaining about what's wrong with the health care system, I was struck by how excited these young people were to enter their new profession.

For some reason, I felt that it was important for me to hit them with a big dose of reality.

"You folks should realize," I began, my voice dripping with gravitas, "that you'll be entering a profession totally unlike the one I entered 30 years ago. You'll be under relentless pressure to figure out how to deliver high quality, safe, satisfying, accessible, equitable care … and do it at the lowest possible cost."

That'll shake the chipper right out of them, I thought.

One bright-eyed young man raised his hand and asked a question that, years later, still makes me chuckle. "What exactly were *you* trying to do?" he asked.

His question, of course, was at once naïve and extraordinarily insightful. It seems self-evident that the health care system—and the policies that govern its structure and conduct—should be organized in a way that delivers the best and least expensive care (today, we'd call this the "highest value care"). And yet any American who has spent more than a few minutes delivering health care, organizing it, or—hardest of all—seeking or receiving it realizes that it is a jury-rigged mess. This is not for lack of resources. In the United States, we spend an inordinate amount of our national wealth ($4.5 trillion per year at last count) on health care, or about 18% of our gross domestic product. Nor is it for lack of good people—by and large, our clinicians and administrators are well trained, smart, ethical, and committed. Yet our outcomes are far from ideal, and the care experience often smacks more of chaos than competence.

"Every system is perfectly designed to deliver the results it delivers," goes the well-worn saying. In order to make sense of the health care system's strengths and deficiencies, it is critical to understand its many moving parts and how they interrelate. The medical, nursing, and pharmacy student focuses on the clinician-patient interaction, and this is as it should be. A vast amount of medical care involves the relationship—bordering on sacred—between a patient seeking help and a clinician trained and duty bound to deliver it.

But we've come to recognize that context matters. A lot. Outside that exam room, and influencing everything that happens inside it, are myriad systems: systems for payment, insurance, regulations, computers, pharmacy, and more. And each of these systems is populated by dozens of players—hospitals, health plans, pharmacy benefits managers, biotech companies, electronic health record vendors, venture capitalists, and many more—each with entrenched interests and particular worldviews. In the end, it is the sum total of these systems and these players that shapes the experience of both patients and clinicians, often determining the experience of not only care but, not uncommonly, life and death.

And these systems and players are anything but static. In 1996, I wrote an article in the *New England Journal of Medicine* in which I coined the term "hospitalist" and made the prediction that this previously unnamed care model—one in which a new breed of generalists would assume the role of coordinator of hospital care—would become a dominant feature of the American health care system.[1] Within a decade, the field of hospital medicine had become the fastest-growing specialty in U.S. medical history. Today, there are more hospitalists, about 60,000, than any other specialty of medicine.

At about the same time, researchers at Johns Hopkins described another new model for hospital care, which they dubbed "hospital at home."[2] Their early studies, which were as rigorous and convincing as the studies supporting the hospitalist model, offered evidence that many hospitalized patients—perhaps 10% to 20%—could be safely cared for at home, at far lower cost and with equal, if not superior, outcomes. Yet 20 years later, thriving hospital at home programs are hard to find (though they now have a little postpandemic wind in their sails).

The example shows that the health care system is capable of not only breathtaking change but also staggering inertia. I remember reading articles from around 1990 talking about how the payment system *had* to change because spending 12% of U.S. gross domestic product was unsustainable. Well, with the fraction now 18%, that prediction was clearly wrong. Similarly, the dominance of value-based care (and the demise of fee-for-service) has been "just around the corner" for more than a quarter-century.

Yet massive change is possible when the stars align. The passage of Obamacare in 2010 resulted in more than 30 million Americans gaining health care insurance coverage. Facilitated by a change in policy and regulations (HITECH and Meaningful Use), while fewer than one-in-ten U.S. hospitals had an electronic health record in 2007, by 2017 fewer than one-in-ten did not. Telemedicine limped along as a futuristic idea until COVID struck, and then it became very real, very quickly.

We're likely on the cusp of even more rapid change, as we come out of a one-in-a-century pandemic and enter an era of rapid technological transformation. Just as technology has changed the way we buy books, access entertainment, manage our money, and interact with the world, it seems clear that health care's technological revolution is finally upon us. With that will come sweeping changes, with tremendous pressures on policymakers to weigh in—sometimes to enable, sometimes to constrain, and sometimes both.

Understanding health policy can seem somewhat divorced from the daily realities of the work of front-line clinicians. And yet it is policy that determines most everything else in the health care system. Since it's about politics, power, passion, and money, it is endlessly fascinating. Since it's also ultimately about people's most prized possession—their health—it's also infinitely important. This book will help you understand it and, I hope, improve it.

Robert M. Wachter, MD
Professor and Chair, Department of Medicine
University of California-San Francisco

References

1. Wachter RM, Goldman L. The emerging role of "hospitalists" in the American health care system. *N Engl J Med.* 1996;335:514-517.
2. Leff B, Burton L, Guido S, Greenough WB, Steinwachs D, Burton JR. Home hospital program: a pilot study. *J Am Geriatr Soc.* 1999;47:697-702.

Four Notes on How to Read This Book

Cross-referencing

There's no way to learn about health systems and policy by starting at Point A and reading steadily and seamlessly until you're at Point Z. Instead, it's like playing Chutes and Ladders, with lots of connections between sections of the path, and trips back and forth between them. To help with those connections, we have cross-referenced topics between sections of the book.

Acronyms

HCIAFOA (Health Care Is a Field of Acronyms). There's no way around it: you're going to have to get familiar with a few. The following acronyms are used frequently throughout the book and, while only spelled out at first in-text reference, will not be repeatedly spelled out. Please refer back to this page if you come across one of these acronyms and forget what it is.

ACA—Affordable Care Act, the 2010 law sometimes also called Obamacare

AHRQ—Agency for Healthcare Research and Quality, the federal agency that evaluates health care services

APM—Alternative Payment Model, also sometimes referred to as Value-Based Care (VBC)

CDC—Centers for Disease Control and Prevention, the federal agency that offers guidance on public health

CMMI—Center for Medicare & Medicaid Innovation, also called the CMS Innovation Center, the part of CMS that pilots new payment and delivery systems

CMS—Centers for Medicare & Medicaid Services, the government service that runs Medicare and Medicaid

ED—Emergency Department

EHR—Electronic Health Records, also sometimes called Electronic Medical Record

ESI—Employer-Sponsored Insurance, getting your insurance through your job

FDA—Food and Drug Administration, the federal agency that regulates pharmaceuticals and devices

FFS—Fee-for-Service, the dominant method of reimbursing for care

GDP—Gross Domestic Product

MA—Medicare Advantage, a privatized form of Medicare

NIH—National Institutes of Health, the federal agency that funds and conducts biomedical research

PBM—Pharmacy Benefits Manager, businesses that act as middlemen between payers and pharmaceutical manufacturers

SDoH—Social Determinants of Health, that is, contributors to health status beyond genetics, pathophysiology, and individual behavior

VA/VHA—Veterans Affairs/Veterans Health Administration, government-run health care for Veterans

Term clarification

Health care is also a field of using a bunch of synonyms and not-quite-synonyms. To make things easier, we are going to clarify what we mean by a few words you'll see throughout the book.

"**Clinician**" refers collectively to physicians, nurse practitioners, and physician assistants. In cases in which we could be referring to this entire group, we will use "clinician." In cases in which we are referring to physicians only, we will use "physician."

"**Provider**" refers to clinicians as well as to larger sources of health services, such as a hospital or a health system.

"**Payer**" refers to whoever is paying for the care. In almost all cases, this is an insurance company, and "payer" can basically be considered synonymous with "insurer" or "insurance company." We use all three terms in this book.

Finally, we want to clarify a few words that are often used interchangeably but are *not* synonyms: **cost, charge, price, reimbursement**, and **spending**. We have tried to be careful to use these precisely throughout the book. See Chapter 3 for more explanation.

Our goals

When we wrote the first edition of this book, we were both medical students, aiming to write the book we ourselves had wanted to read. Before medical school, and during it, we had tried to cobble together an understanding of what health care even was. We found ourselves lost in a sea of confusion, faced with specialized publications that didn't seem to add up to a coherent whole. So we decided to write the book we wanted to read.

Our goal with this book is to provide a broad base of facts, concepts, and analysis so the reader gets a thorough overview of the American health care system—and a jumping-off point from which to learn more in their areas of interest and develop their own opinions. Our goal is to give a readable, engaging big picture overview, dipping into the details when interesting or necessary. Since nuance and brevity don't usually go hand in hand, at times we had to make concessions on one side or the other.

And, finally, our goal is to impress upon the reader how complicated these issues are. This stuff is complex, solutions get thwarted by reality, and understanding one issue means you have to read about three other issues first. It's always more complicated than you think!

Introduction:
The Lay of the Land

It's beyond the scope of this book to talk about the health care systems of other nations—we've got our hands full with this one!—but we need to at least make a few comparisons. After all, you can analyze the performance of an Olympic figure skater all day, but it's not until you get a sense of the competition that you can really understand her skills and faults. While skaters are judged on their skills, composition, and interpretation of music, health systems are judged on cost, access, and quality. Let's take a look at how we compare to some of our peer nations.

Cost

The United States spends nearly 20% of its national gross domestic product (GDP) on health care, far more than any other country in the world. Health care spending now averages over $12,500 per American,[1] and health care is the largest and fastest-growing industry in the country[2] (see Figure 1[3]).

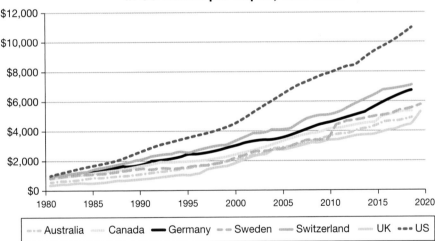

Comparison of Health Spending of Selected Countries, in US Dollars per Capita, 1980-2020

Figure 1 Source: Data from OECD. *Health Spending* (indicator). OECD Publishing; 2022. Accessed April 25, 2022. doi:10.1787/8643de7e-en

Access

Access can be defined in several ways (as we'll get to later in the book). But the United States has fewer physicians and hospital beds per capita than most other peer nations.[4] And while 90% of Americans report having a regular source of ongoing care, the United States does poorly on affordability and timeliness of that care (Figure 2).[5] There are also large disparities in access depending on the type of health insurance coverage.

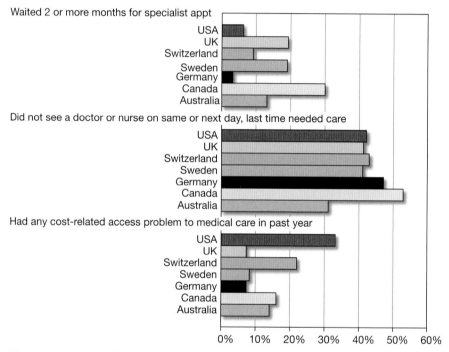

Figure 2 Source: Osborn R, Squires D, Doty MM, Sarnak DO, Schneider EC. In new survey of eleven countries, US adults still struggle with access to and affordability of health care. *Health Aff (Millwood)*. 2016;35(12):2327-2336. doi:10.1377/hlthaff.2016.1088

Quality

Despite spending all that money, we don't have the best health outcomes. Our burden of disease is higher, postoperative complications and errors are more common, and maternal mortality rates are high and rising (particularly for Black women).[6] On the bright side, we're generally improving on all those measures, plus our cancer survival rates are near the top.[7] Unfortunately, our already low rankings for avoidable mortality and life expectancy at birth both worsened during the pandemic[8] (see Figure 3[9]).

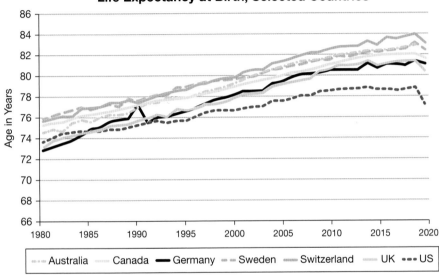

Figure 3   Source: Data from OECD. *Life Expectancy at Birth* (indicator). OECD Publishing; 2022. Accessed April 25, 2022. doi:10.1787/27e0fc9d-en

Summary

The most recent major international comparison by the Commonwealth Fund ranked our system 11th—which isn't so bad … until you realize that the study only included 11 countries (see Table 1[10]).

Any way you slice it, the U.S. health care system has room for improvement. Now let's jump in and examine the details.[11]

Table 1 Health Care System Performance Rankings, 2021

	AUS	CAN	FRA	GER	NET	NZ	NOR	SWE	SWZ	UK	US
Overall	3	10	8	5	2	6	1	7	9	4	**11**
Access	8	9	7	3	1	5	2	6	10	4	**11**
Care Process	6	4	10	9	3	1	8	11	7	5	**2**
Admin Efficiency	2	7	6	9	8	3	1	5	10	4	**11**
Equity	1	10	7	2	5	9	8	6	3	4	**11**
Outcomes	1	10	6	7	4	8	2	5	3	9	**11**

Source: Schneider EC, Shah A, Doty MM, Tikkanen R, Fields K, Williams II RD. Mirror, Mirror 2021: Reflecting Poorly—Health Care in the U.S. Compared to Other High-Income Countries. Commonwealth Fund; August 4, 2021. doi:10.26099/01dv-h208

References

1. Centers for Medicare and Medicaid Services. *NHE Fact Sheet*. 2021. Accessed April 26, 2022. https://www.cms.gov/Research-Statistics-Data-and-Systems/Statistics-Trends-and-Reports/NationalHealthExpendData/NHE-Fact-Sheet

2. Bureau of Labor Statistics. *Occupational Outlook Handbook*. 2022.

3. Data from OECD. *Health Spending* (indicator). OECD Publishing; 2022. Accessed April 25, 2022. doi:10.1787/8643de7e-en

4. OECD. Indicator overview: country dashboards and major trends. In: *Health at a Glance 2021: OECD Indicators*. OECD Publishing; 2021.

5. Schneider EC, Shah A, Doty MM, Tikkanen R, Fields K, Williams II RD. *Mirror, Mirror 2021: Reflecting Poorly—Health Care in the U.S. Compared to Other High-Income Countries*. Commonwealth Fund; August 4, 2021. doi:10.26099/01dv-h208

6. 2021 National Healthcare Quality and Disparities Report. AHRQ Pub. No. 21(22)-0054-EF. Agency for Healthcare Research and Quality; December 2021.

7. OECD. *Cancer Care: Assuring Quality to Improve Survival*. OECD Health Policy Studies. OECD Publishing; 2013. doi:10.1787/9789264181052-en

8. OECD. *Health at a Glance 2021: OECD Indicators*. OECD Publishing; 2021. doi:10.1787/ae3016b9-en

9. Data from OECD. *Life Expectancy at Birth* (indicator). OECD Publishing; 2022. Accessed April 25, 2022. doi:10.1787/27e0fc9d-en

10. Osborn R, Squires D, Doty MM, Sarnak DO, Schneider EC. In new survey of eleven countries, US adults still struggle with access to and affordability of health care. *Health Aff (Millwood)*. 2016;35(12): 2327-2336. doi:10.1377/hlthaff.2016.1088

11. Schneider EC, Shah A, Doty MM, Tikkanen R, Fields K, Williams II RD. *Mirror, Mirror 2021: Reflecting Poorly—Health Care in the U.S. Compared to Other High-Income Countries*. Commonwealth Fund; August 4, 2021. doi:10.26099/01dv-h208

Acknowledgments

First and foremost, we want to thank our extremely patient, supportive, and incredible spouses, David Askin and Osamuede Osemwota, whom we are very lucky to have. We also thank our kids, who have forgiven us that this book is about health care rather than wizards or talking trains.

Second, we thank Joe Cho, Maria McAvey, and everyone on the Wolters Kluwer team. We also thank our research interns, Tamara Sanchez-Ortiz and Victoria Chi.

Our deepest gratitude goes to the senior physicians and leaders who have mentored and supported us with this book. We particularly thank Dr William Peck from Washington University School of Medicine and Dr Bob Wachter from the University of California-San Francisco.

Least, but not last, we thank the many folks kind enough to read our drafts and offer knowledgeable, useful, and engaging feedback. Endless thanks to Jay Albertina, Chuck Askin, Punita Bhansali, Tom Byrne, Aaron Baird, Brian Carter, Arvan Chan, John Corker, Ben Cutone, Jennifer Dellazanna, Randall Ellis, Tommy Emmet, Eric Epping, Jesse Favre, John Goodson, Kelbe Goupil, Julia Halterman, Zoë Leigh Heins, Sims Hershey, Leslie Jackson, Jenny Ji, Karen Joynt Maddox, Omair Khan, Emmeline Kim, Caroline Kimberly, Pam King, Andrea Kjos, Sterling Lee, Abby Leibowitz, Nidhish Lokesh, Christopher Loumeau, Walter Markowitz, Mark Mayer, Alec McCranie, Angela Mihalic, Aman Narayan, David Newton, Oluwatomi Oluwasanmi, Charlene Palton, Andrew Pierce, Georgia Rae-Jones, Omar Samara, John Schutz, Heather Shafter, Dale Tager, Avi Tutman, Erik Wallace, Amber Weydert, and Richelle Williams.

A Note on the Inflation Reduction Act

The Inflation Reduction Act (IRA) was passed by Congress and signed into law in August 2022, 4 months after the manuscript for this book was turned in, but a few months before printing. Health policy changes constantly, and we mostly have to resign ourselves to going out of date the moment we turn in our manuscript. In this case, however, the IRA is the most important health legislation since the passing of the Affordable Care Act in 2010, and we want to make sure to address it.

Here is a brief summary of the IRA's major health provisions, which primarily affect Medicare patients in Part D prescription drug coverage plans:

Protections for Medicare patients

- Places a $35 cap on monthly copays for insulin. Insulin payments will stay the same, but Medicare will shield patients from it (as of 2023).
- Places a $2,000 annual cap on out-of-pocket drug spending and limits how much premiums can rise each year in Part D prescription drug plans. (Some limits start in 2023, with a full cap as of 2025.)

Regulation of pharmaceutical companies

- Charge rebates to pharmaceutical companies for drug prices that rise faster than inflation (as of 2023).
- Requires Medicare to negotiate reimbursements for a limited number of pharmaceutical drugs each year, starting with 10 drugs in 2026 and increasing to 20 by 2029. This is a complicated policy, with lots of exclusions as well as a complex structure for negotiations.
- Redesigns Part D coverage, removing responsibility for coverage of high expenditures from patients entirely, and shifting the bulk of the responsibility from mostly Medicare to mostly the Part D private plans and manufacturers themselves (as of 2025).

For a description of Medicare Part D, see Section "Medicare" in Chapter 2. For a description of how pharmaceutical drugs are paid for, Section "Paying for Prescription Drugs" in Chapter 5. For a discussion of the controversy over drug costs and Medicare negotiating that cost, see Section "Drug Pricing Controversies" in Chapter 5.

For more information about the health provisions of the IRA, we recommend Kaiser Family Foundation (always!), as well as the August 10, 2022, Health Affairs Forefront Article "Understanding the Democrats' Drug Pricing Package" by Rachel Sachs.

Contents

1

Systems and Delivery

Questions as you read through the chapter:

1. What does it mean to deliver health care in America—what is being delivered, where, and by whom?
2. What are the options for how to get care, and what barriers stand in the way?
3. Is care delivered in an equitable way in the United States? What might make it more equitable? Who should determine or incentivize those changes?
4. How should the delivery system incorporate home-based care?
5. In what ways is care delivery the same as it was 50 years ago? Ten years ago? In what ways is it different? What is positive or negative about those changes?

We all experience aspects of health and illness every day, but most of us live our lives outside of a medical setting. And when you hear about medical care, you might think of the doctors and nurses in the TV shows *Scrubs* or *Grey's Anatomy*, both of which are set in teaching hospitals, yet the majority of care is delivered outside of such intense settings.

In the 1960s, researchers aimed to describe the landscape of illness and care delivery across a community. Their report, called the *Ecology of Medical Care*, described, out of 1,000 people in a given month, how many had health symptoms and how many got care in a clinic, at home, in an ER, or in a hospital. Forty years later, that study was updated and, despite a world changed by medical innovations, it found much the same breakdown in the number of people getting the same types of care.[1,2]

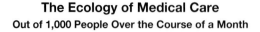

The Ecology of Medical Care
Out of 1,000 People Over the Course of a Month

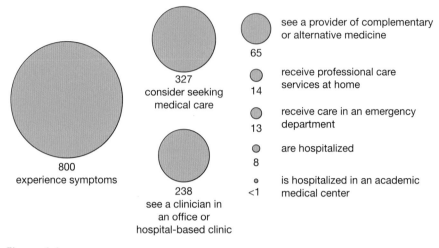

327
consider seeking
medical care

800
experience symptoms

238
see a clinician in
an office or
hospital-based clinic

65   see a provider of complementary or alternative medicine

14   receive professional care services at home

13   receive care in an emergency department

8   are hospitalized

<1   is hospitalized in an academic medical center

Figure 1.1

It might seem funny to use the word "ecology"—a biology term—to refer to the provision of medical services in an advanced society, but the term is very appropriate for care delivery because it evokes a wild ecosystem that developed organically rather than a planned system. We will use this term as well as the breakdown in Figure 1.1 as a framework in this chapter to understand the delivery of care in America. (See Chapter 7 for *who* delivers the care.)

Even though the smallest elements—hospitalization—of our *Ecology* diagram serve the fewest people, they are where the disproportionate share of resources, funding, and health care workers are devoted, so that's where we'll start. We'll follow the path a patient might take, from getting to the hospital (using an ambulance and the emergency department [ED]), being in the hospital, and then going to a nursing facility afterward. Once we've discussed this path, we'll zoom out, to look at outpatient care, then home care, and then finally public and population health, which aim to promote the health of all 1,000 people in our ecology.

Getting to the Hospital

Emergency Medical Services and Ambulances

Most emergency medical services are accredited by the government but run by private agencies. In 2020, about 18,200 agencies—employing a million trained personnel (see Section "Emergency Medical Technician/Paramedic [EMT]" in Chapter 7)—supplied ambulance rides, first responders for medical emergencies, and emergency air flight services.[3] They responded to 28 million 911 calls and made 190,000 airlifts. For an ambulance ride, a typical charge is around $1,000—a cost not always covered by insurance.[4]

The ER ... or ED ("Emergency Department") ... or EU ("Emergency Unit")

We'll go with ED. Whatever acronym you use, the ED is a well-known and essential place for medical care. It is an option for people who cannot access care anywhere else, because they don't have a primary doctor, their doctor's office is closed, they are traveling, or they cannot afford to go anywhere else. Most EDs are very busy places. They are legally required to evaluate all patients regardless of ability to pay (see Emergency Medical Treatment and Active Labor Act [EMTALA] in Section "Timeline of Major Public Health and Health Policy Developments" in Chapter 6), see an incredible range of medical problems (Table 1.1), and sometimes don't get reimbursed.

EDs are technically defined as "outpatient" rather than "inpatient" (ie, hospital) services, but they are typically physically connected to (and vital for) hospitals because they serve as a major point of entry for hospital admissions. (Patients can also bypass the ED to be "directly" admitted to the hospital, though, for instance, after a planned surgery.)

Fast facts:

- There were 130 million estimated ED visits in 2018.[5]
- The average expenditure on an ED visit in 2017 was $1,016.[6]
- The highest ED visit rates are by infants less than 1 year old, adults over age 75, women, non-Hispanic Black patients, and patients on Medicaid.[7]
- Of all patients seen in 2014, an average of 14% were admitted to the hospital.[8]
- 17% of ED visits include a computed tomography (CT) scan.[9]

Table 1.1 Top Five Problems Seen in Emergency Departments (EDs), 2014

Abdominal problems (pain, vomiting, etc)	11.8%
Mental health and substance use	4.5%
Upper respiratory infections	4.2%
Sprains and strains	4.1%
Chest pain	4.1%

Source: Hooker EA, Mallow PJ, Oglesby MM. Characteristics and trends of emergency department visits in the United States (2010-2014). *J Emerg Med*. 2019;56(3):344-351. doi:10.1016/j.jemermed.2018.12.025

Hospital or Inpatient Care

A hospital provides "acute" care, meaning you need immediate medical and nursing care and observation and cannot wait for an appointment. Generally, a hospital is a facility where a person stays overnight and is taken care of by multiple health professionals (but definitely at least a nurse and a clinician). There are 6,090 hospitals in the United States (Figure 1.2), with nearly a million beds, employing 6.6 million workers,[10] and caring for over 36 million patients a year.[11] Let's take a bird's-eye view.

Take a look at the map in Figure 1.3. Notice there are more blue dots where there are more people. You cannot just go out and open a hospital—or even a specialized center within a hospital—anywhere you want. Since 1964, most states have Certificate of Need (CON) laws, meaning that any creation, expansion, or purchase of a health care facility has to be approved by state regulators. The purpose of such laws is to ensure access for underserved communities, constrain costs, and ensure that hospitals focus on needed care and are not just another flashy cardiac surgery center designed to entice rich patients. However, many feel CON laws haven't served their purpose,[12] and most were suspended or repealed during the COVID-19 pandemic—when rapidly filling hospitals didn't exactly have time to ask permission to add hospital beds.[13]

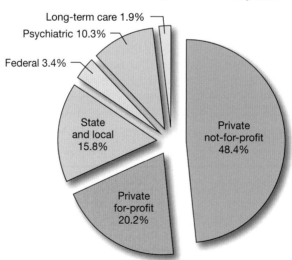

Breakdown of 6,090 U.S. Hospitals

Long-term care 1.9%
Psychiatric 10.3%
Federal 3.4%
State and local 15.8%
Private for-profit 20.2%
Private not-for-profit 48.4%

Figure 1.2 Used with permission of American Hospital Association.

Types of Hospitals

Public

County (or Local): Most public hospitals are safety-net, general hospitals that maintain a primary focus on caring for underserved populations. In 2021, there were 962 state and local hospitals.[11] Examples: Cook County Hospital in Chicago, Parkland Memorial Hospital in Dallas.

State: State hospitals are typically long-term facilities for psychiatric patients.

Federal: Three federal government agencies operate hospitals—the Department of Defense for active military members (32 hospitals[14]), the Indian Health Service (IHS) for Native Americans (46 hospitals[15]), and the Veterans Health Administration (170 hospitals[16]) for military veterans.

Prisons: Prison hospitals are administered by federal, state, or local governments or by private contractors. Medical services account for about a fifth of all prison expenditures.[17]

Private (or Community) Hospitals

Private or community hospitals are those not operated by the government. However, most hospitals cannot afford *not* to take Medicare insurance (because Medicare is the single largest insurer in the United States), and so are in some sense *funded* by the government. There is a huge amount of variability in community hospitals; they might be general (ie, offer many different types of services) or specialty (ie, focus on one type of service or population, such as obstetrics or orthopedic surgery), they might be for-profit or not-for-profit, and they might include academic research and training as a major component of their mission.

A few prominent types

Not-for-Profit: Not-for-profit institutions, particularly religious ones, are mainstays that historically stem from charity institutions for the poor. Profit is reinvested in the hospital or community, rather than given to shareholders. These hospitals typically maintain a commitment to charity care, although this is often not their primary focus. Some not-for-profit hospitals function as safety-net hospitals; recognizing the community benefit of the charity care not-for-profit hospitals provide, the government doesn't require these hospitals to pay taxes.[a,4]

Academic Medical Centers: The United States has over 1,000 teaching hospitals.[18] They're connected with medical schools, have residency programs (see Section "Graduate Medical Education" in Chapter 7), and patients there are likely to see both students and residents, as these

---

[a]Though we should note the difference between a "not-for-profit" and a "charity care" hospital. They overlap but are not the same.

Map of Community Hospitals in the United States

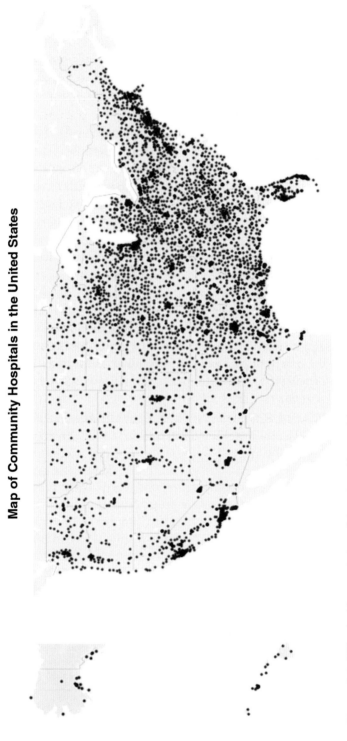

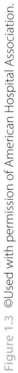

Figure 1.3 ©Used with permission of American Hospital Association.

institutions explicitly include the training of health care professionals as part of their mission. They're often large hospitals located in major urban centers and provide a significant amount of charity care (note that residency programs are very frequently affiliated with county and VA hospitals, too). Example: Cleveland Clinic in Cleveland.

Religious: Many religious organizations have opened hospitals over the years, seeking to serve their own population, the underserved, or the community at large. Religious hospitals make up 18.5% of all hospitals in the United States, and most of these are Catholic.[19] The direct impact of the religious organization on the day-to-day management of the hospital varies; in one arrangement, religious leaders comprise a portion of the board of directors, but a lay CEO oversees hospital operations. Example: Loma Linda Medical Center in Los Angeles.

Children's: These may be general hospitals for children or they may be a section of a medical–surgical hospital. There are over 250 children's hospitals in the United States,[20] many of which also serve as teaching and research institutions. Example: Children's Hospital of Philadelphia.

For-Profit: For-profit hospitals are owned by private corporations, and some of the hospital's profit is given to shareholders (as opposed to all of it being reinvested into operations). Unlike not-for-profit hospitals, these organizations are required to pay taxes. The largest operator of for-profit hospitals is the Hospital Corporation of America, which owns and operates 184 hospitals across the country.[21]

Physician-Owned Hospitals: As of 2020, the United States had about 250 physician-owned hospitals.[22] The majority are for-profit institutions, and they are all limited in expansion by the Affordable Care Act (ACA). These hospitals can be of any type but are more likely to be single specialty—especially orthopedics, oncology, or cardiology—than hospitals that don't have physician owners.[23]

Hospital Networks

Most hospitals—nearly 70%—do not operate in isolation but are part of a system or network,[11] an organization that owns and operates multiple hospitals and/or outpatient facilities (see Section "The (Big) Business of Medicine" in Chapter 3) (Figure 1.4).

Hospital Operations

In 2021, U.S. hospitals had over $1 trillion in expenses.[11] This means a hospital is a big business, and operating one is just as complex, if not more so, than operating any other large corporation.

Health System Size, by Ownership Type, 2018

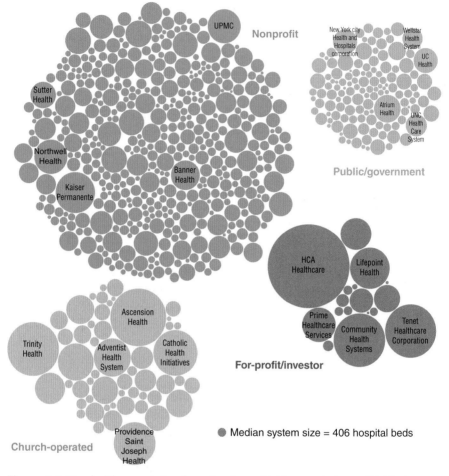

Figure 1.4 Used with permission from Furukawa M, Kimmey L, Jones DJ, Machta RM, Guo J, Rich E. Consolidation and health systems in 2018: new data from the AHRQ Compendium. Accessed November 25, 2019. https://www.healthaffairs.org/do/10.1377/forefront.20191122.345861/full/

A general hospital contains units of different types of care, including the ED, the intensive care unit (ICU), and general ward, as well as more specialized units such as the postanesthesia care unit (PACU) and labor and delivery ward. They care for a huge variety of conditions, with labor and delivery being the most common, and serious infection ("sepsis") being the second[24] (Figure 1.5).

In addition, far more people make the hospital run than just the clinicians a patient sees. Types of services include administrators (like quality assurance officers), therapeutic (physicians, nurses, pharmacists, physical therapists,

Aggregate Cost of Hospital Inpatient Stays, Top 10 Diagnoses, 2018

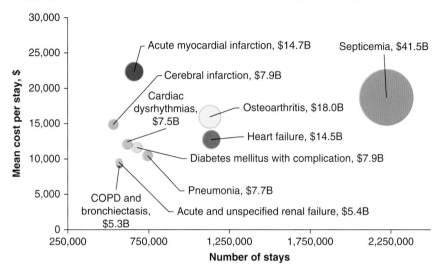

Figure 1.5 B, billion; COPD, chronic obstructive pulmonary disease; ICD-10-CM, International Classification of Diseases, Tenth Revision, Clinical Modification. Notes: Excludes maternal and neonatal admissions. Diagnoses were identified using the Clinical Classifications Software Refined (CCSR) for ICD-10-CM diagnoses. The pneumonia diagnosis group excludes pneumonia caused by tuberculosis. (From McDermott KW, Roemer M. Most frequent principal diagnoses for inpatient stays in U.S. Hospitals, 2018. HCUP Statistical Brief #277. Agency for Healthcare Research and Quality. July 2021. https://www.hcup-us.ahrq.gov/reports/statbriefs/sb277-Top-Reasons-Hospital-Stays-2018.pdf)

etc), diagnostic (lab and radiology technicians), informational (such as coders and information technologists), and support (such as cafeteria servers and janitors). Hospitals are often major employers in their regions.

What are the major considerations for hospitals in delivering care? Things like:

- What are the predominant conditions we care for, and how do we optimize our operations for those specific needs? The needs of a labor and delivery ward are very different from an organ transplant unit.
- How many beds do we have, how do we fit nursing staff availability to those beds, and how do we plan for being nimble in a surge? (Particularly relevant during the COVID-19 pandemic, especially with loss of staff to isolation and quarantine.)
- How do we set up workflows so that patients can flow from one part of their hospitalization to the next, ensuring there won't be a bottleneck at leaving the ED, for instance?

■ How do we ensure quick action when needed, such as a massive transfusion protocol for someone who is losing lots of blood, which involves efficiently coordinating multiple separate therapeutic and diagnostic services?

Most operations are motivated by an aim to provide high-quality care. However, what delivery of care looks like can be very intertwined with how that care is reimbursed. Medicare reimbursement policy, in particular, can steer operations, because (a) Medicare is the largest insurer in the United States, and (b) many private payers will match Medicare policies. Over the decades, Medicare has made a number of changes in their payment policy in order to decrease spending on inpatient care; hospitals will respond to such changes to continue maximizing revenue as best as they can. In one high-profile example, in 2013, Medicare stopped paying higher inpatient rates for hospital care unless a patient stayed at least two midnights in the hospital. (Hospitals can label a patient's care as being "outpatient," "inpatient," or "observation" status—the care can be the same but the label is different.) Hospitals were incentivized to avoid admitting patients for short stays—but, notoriously, they partially responded not by avoiding admissions but rather by simply labeling the patient's stay differently, as "observation" rather than "inpatient" status.[25] Delivery did change—but not as expected. For a second high-profile example, in 2010, Medicare began penalizing hospitals for readmissions within 30 days after discharge for certain conditions. In this case, most hospitals did develop substantial new programs attempting to prevent patients from needing to come back to the hospital once they left it. Nearly all hospitals shifted their operations to focus on discharge planning. In this case, the payment policy definitely reduced Medicare spending and definitely affected operations—but the impact on quality of care has been less clear. Please see the Case Study on Hospital Readmissions at the end of this book.

Post-acute Care

Patients can go to multiple places when they leave the hospital. About 11% of hospital inpatients, who are well enough to leave the hospital but not yet well enough to be home, will be discharged to post-acute care[26] (Figure 1.6). Post-acute care—the umbrella term for skilled nursing facilities (SNFs), long-term acute care hospitals, and inpatient rehabilitation facilities—isn't mentioned in the *Ecology of Medical Care*, but such facilities are a very important aspect of resource allocation and spending. (Distinctions get confusing here, so let's clarify that post-acute care is different from long-term nursing care, like in a nursing home where someone lives permanently, or from care someone gets in their own home.)[26]

Skilled Nursing Facilities: These provide 24-hour nursing care, physical rehabilitation, and assistance with activities of daily living (ie, cooking, eating,

Discharge Location of Inpatient Stays, 2013

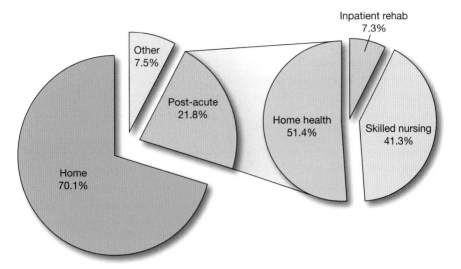

Figure 1.6 Adapted from Tian W. (AHRQ). An all-payer view of hospital discharge to postacute care, 2013. HCUP Statistical Brief #205. Agency for Healthcare Research and Quality. May 2016. http://www.hcup-us.ahrq.gov/reports/statbriefs/sb205-Hospital-Discharge-Postacute-Care.pdf

bathing). As of 2017, there were 15,090 SNFs.[27] Stays can be as brief as 3 days, although Medicare will (partially) cover up to 100 days.

Long-Term Acute Care Hospitals: These serve patients who need intensive, hospital-level care for weeks or months, such as for someone on a ventilator. Patients in these hospitals typically have multiple, complex medical problems. In 2020, there were 348 in the United States[28]

Inpatient Rehab Facilities: Also known as acute rehabilitation hospitals, these facilities care for patients who require comprehensive physical and oc-cupational therapy but not as much nursing care. Patients often enter these fa-cilities after strokes, serious fractures, or joint replacement surgeries. In 2017, there were 1,180 in the United States.[27]

Home Health: Home Health is discussed further in Section "Home Health and Home-Based Care." For short-term needs, Medicare will pay for nurses, phys-ical therapists, occupational therapists, social workers, and aides to come to a patient's home after a hospitalization or major event, as long as their clinician documents that leaving the home would be taxing or impossible. This is only intermittent care, such as seeing a nurse twice a week.

In the past decade, post-acute care has received heightened policy attention because of high spending—over $62 billion a year from Medicare alone[29]—and this attention only sharpened during the COVID-19 pandemic. Given room-sharing, high staff turnover, and sicker, older patients at high risk for infection, these facilities were high-profile locations of outbreaks and deaths. In order to improve post-acute care, policy-makers focus on issues like staff turnover (very high[30]; see Figure 1.7), funding (organizations operate at tiny profit margins, or even losses[31]), and quality reporting.[30]

Outpatient or "Ambulatory" Care

Outpatient care is often referred to as "ambulatory" care, the idea being that you can walk in (and hopefully out) on your own. Outpatient visits may include minor surgery, checkups, physical therapy, mammograms, and lab testing, to name a few examples. Compare the 8 patients hospitalized, in the *Ecology of Medical Care*, to the 238 who see a clinician and 65 who see an

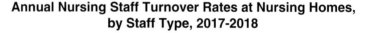

Annual Nursing Staff Turnover Rates at Nursing Homes, by Staff Type, 2017-2018

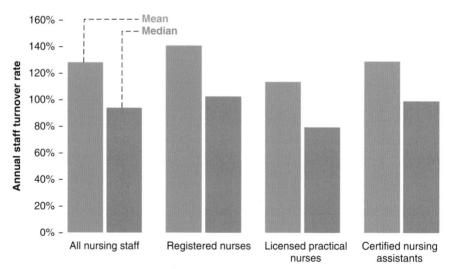

Figure 1.7 The Centers for Medicare and Medicaid Services (CMS) publishes public comparative quality data through Nursing Home Compare, and anyone can look these up at https://www.medicare.gov/care-compare/ (see Chapter 4). Source: Author's analysis of data from the Payroll-Based Journal. Notes: Annual turnover rates are measured as a percentage of the hours of nursing care that a facility provides. We calculated the turnover rate by summing the percentages of care hours provided by departing employees in the 90 days before their last workday. (Adapted from Gandhi A, Yu H, Grabowski DC. High nursing staff turnover in nursing homes offers important quality information. *Health Aff (Millwood)*. 2021;40(3):384-391. doi:10.1377/hlthaff.2020.00957)

alternative health practitioner. In 2016, there were nearly 900,000 office visits to a physician,[32] 54% of those to primary care[32] and 37% for a chronic condition.[33] Interestingly, despite the bulk of care happening in the outpatient setting, relatively few registered nurses are employed in ambulatory settings (only 18%, compared to 60% in the hospital[34]).

Some medical care can be provided in either the inpatient or the outpatient setting. Because of convenience and lower cost, when possible, that care is delivered in the outpatient setting. There is a trend to make some outpatient settings better able to provide robust care: for example, going to urgent care instead of the ER for a broken arm, or having a knee replacement in an ambulatory surgery center (ASC) instead of at the hospital.[b]

In this section, we will look at some of the major types of facilities, services, and organizations common in outpatient care, keeping in mind that patients may get their care from one or more types. There are other, less common types of care practices, such as employer-based clinics, not discussed here.

Types of Clinics

Private Practice

A private practice is an outpatient clinic owned and operated by the health care professionals who practice there. Private practices are often classified in two ways: solo or group, single specialty or multispecialty. Private practice has historically been the dominant form of outpatient care in the United States, but the model is dying out, mostly in favor of hospital- or network-affiliated practices (see Section "The (Big) Business of Medicine" in Chapter 3). Some remaining private practice clinics are transitioning to what's called *direct primary care* or *concierge* care. Concierge practices focus on patients who want a high level of service (eg, short wait times, long appointments, and physicians who are available 24/7) and are willing to pay for it. These practices typically do not bill insurance but instead charge an annual membership fee, sometimes along with separate appointment fees, and can therefore afford to keep the total patient load low and have more time for each patient. Note, however, that these patients still would need insurance for any care not provided in the office.

Hospital- or Network-Affiliated Practice

In many cases, a primary care or specialty clinic might be started—or a private group practice will be purchased—by a hospital or health care network. These clinicians may be integrated into normal hospital operations, be housed in a

---

[b]Some centers now even offer "hospital at home" programs where inpatients remain at home while the nurses, clinicians, medications, etc, come to the house.

separate section of the building, or practice in traditional community-based locations. From the point of view of a patient, these clinics function very similarly to a private practice, but they tend to be better integrated with other doctors or hospitals within a network, and the clinicians are employees rather than owners. Technically, this category includes the networked federal clinics in the VA (1,063 clinics[16]) and TRICARE (373 clinics[14]).

Community Health Centers/Federally Qualified Health Centers

These are government-supported clinics that provide low-cost care to underserved and low-income populations. Community health centers (CHCs) often focus on primary care but may offer a range of services in a "one-stop shop" format. For instance, some offer laboratory testing, obstetrics/gynecology, behavioral health, pharmacy, and dental services in addition to primary care. In 2020, more than 14,500 CHCs were providing care to 28 million patients annually.[35]

Nearly 1,400 CHCs are also designated as federally qualified health centers (FQHCs),[36] which enables them to receive extra funding from Medicare, Medicaid, and Children's Health Insurance Program (CHIP). This category includes clinics through the IHS (433 clinics[15]). Beyond CHCs, there are also a variety of "free clinics" caring for small numbers of underserved and low-income populations. Free clinics tend to be funded and operated by private not-for-profit organizations.

Urgent Care Center

There are about 8,700 urgent care centers (UCCs)[37] bridging the gap between primary care and the ED. They're open on evenings and weekends, appealing to patients who can't get same-day appointments, need medical care outside of normal office hours, or don't have regular primary care physicians. However, UCCs aren't equipped to deal with trauma or emergencies. Common services offered by UCCs are laceration and fracture care, x-rays, school and employment physicals, and immunizations. During the COVID-19 pandemic, UCCs were an important source of respiratory care and testing.[38]

Beyond UCCs, the past decade has seen rapid growth in retail clinics, located in convenient locations (for instance, there are over 1,100 CVS MinuteClinics[39]) offering quick, inexpensive, protocol-based care for limited medical conditions, such as strep throat, minor burns, and basic preventive health testing like cholesterol. Patients who present with urgent or more complicated conditions are referred to EDs, UCCs, or other local physicians.

Ambulatory Surgery Center

Although surgical services are often closely linked with hospitals, more than 60% of surgical procedures in the United States do not require an overnight stay.[40] ASCs are separate from hospitals and operate like surgical clinics for same-day procedures. The most common procedures performed at the 9,280 ASCs[41] in the United States are colonoscopies, endoscopies, and cataract removals.[42] There is a trend toward including more complex procedures in ASCs, including joint replacements, particularly as insurers—like Medicare—adjust payment policy to reduce high inpatient spending. Nearly all ASCs are owned at least in part by physicians.[43]

Dialysis Centers

About half a million people in the United States have end-stage renal disease (ESRD) requiring long-term dialysis to live.[44] Dialysis typically lasts 3 to 4 hours at a time, and most people need three treatments per week. As you might imagine, then, the 7,400 dialysis centers nationwide are the central point of connection to the health system for patients with ESRD.[44] About 70% of dialysis centers are owned by two chains: DaVita and Fresenius.[45]

Nonphysician Services

Dentists, chiropractors, podiatrists, physical therapists, and optometrists are just a few of the professionals who practice primarily in outpatient settings. Further, nearly half of Americans[46] regularly use complementary (used with conventional medicine) or alternative (used in place of conventional medicine) therapies, which include herbal or natural products, acupuncture, and homeopathic care. Although major insurers will pay for some of these services, much is out of pocket (for instance, nearly half of Medicare beneficiaries do not have dental insurance,[47] and Americans spend over $14 billion out of pocket annually on complementary and alternative medicine[48]).

Pharmacies

Pharmacies aren't mentioned in the *Ecology of Medical Care*, but they are indispensable in many people's lives and to the delivery system. As a business, pharmacies buy and sell medications. As a clinical service, pharmacists do much more: checking for correct prescription orders (clinicians make more mistakes than you'd think), ensuring a medication won't cause harmful effects because of certain medical conditions or drug interactions, and teaching patients about safe medication usage. Increasingly, pharmacies also provide care traditionally given in doctor's offices, like vaccinations.

An interesting news story to underscore the clinical role and responsibility of pharmacists is that pharmacies are getting some blame for the opioid epidemic. In late 2021, a jury in Ohio found Walgreens, CVS, and Walmart pharmacies partially liable for the opioid epidemic[49] (see Section "The Opioid Epidemic" in Chapter 6). Such a judgment may be surprising, but it also reflects the importance of every element of the delivery system in determining health outcomes.

There are about 67,000 community pharmacies in the United States, most of which are either independently owned or run by a retail chain like Walgreens (Figure 1.8).[50] Pharmacies purchase their medications from manufacturers and deal with business woes common to the delivery system: high drug prices, low margins, tough negotiations with pharmacy benefits managers (PBMs), and corporate consolidation (see Section "The (Big) Business of Medicine" on PBMs in Chapter 3, and Section "Paying for Prescriptions Drugs" in Chapter 5). Sometimes these issues lead to closures, and an estimated 40% of counties are "pharmacy deserts,"[51] where people must drive more than 15 minutes to reach a pharmacy. Pharmacy deserts are usually rural but can affect urban areas, such as San Francisco, where the southeastern neighborhoods, which have the highest prevalence of low-income households and highest concentration of Black and Latino residents, only have a single pharmacy to serve 35,000 people.[52] This issue can be—and increasingly is—addressed by mail-order pharmacies, often run by PBMs, such as Express Scripts.[53]

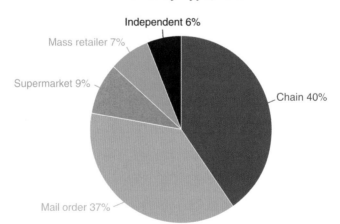

Market Share of Retail Prescription Drug Sales by Pharmacy Type, 2017

Independent 6%
Mass retailer 7%
Supermarket 9%
Chain 40%
Mail order 37%

Figure 1.8 Data: Retail pharmacy sales data from IQVIA and National Association of Chain Drug Stores, *Chair Member Fact Book 2018-2019* (NACDS, May 2019), 55. (Adapted from Seeley E, Singh S. Competition, consolidation, and evolution in the pharmacymarket: implications for efforts to contain drug prices and spending. *Commonwealth Fund.* 2021. doi:10.26099/exwh-r479)

Telemedicine and Telehealth

Telemedicine—which technically encompasses both telephone and video visits, but really is more about video visits, which are reimbursed at higher rates than telephone visits—was barely a blip before the COVID-19 pandemic. Although some video and virtual care began before the pandemic (particularly by the Veterans Health Administration to reach rural veterans), video visits for traditional primary and specialty care didn't hit mainstream until March 2020. Because of the preferences and requirements for distancing during the pandemic, as well as the scarcity of personal protective equipment, most clinics rapidly transitioned to virtual care for most patients. Across the nation, 0.1% of Medicare primary care appointments were conducted by video in February 2020; 2 months later, 43.5% were.[54] The use of video even extended to the hospital—allowing care teams to talk to actively infected patients without repeat exposures in the room, allowing patients to see loved ones when visitors were barred, and even allowing physicians from far away to help when New York City hospitals were overloaded.

Video visits can serve patients well, removing the need to take half a day off work, and allowing a visit even when you have trouble getting to the clinic or are out of town.[c] They will likely remain a significant proportion of all outpatient visits. In fact, by late 2020, all health centers were conducting 30% of visits virtually.[55] The shift to widespread telemedicine is a major one. Much of medical care through history has centered around the physical presence of the patient: the physical exam, state medical licensing, gathering data (such as vital signs and lab tests), and, last but not least, reimbursement. Logistics have improved with the electronic era (your doctor can send a lab order or prescription to a far-away location electronically), but some questions will take time to work out—like what problems warrant a physical exam, and whether it makes sense to keep licensing clinicians by state rather than nationally (see Section "Licensing—Approval by the (State) Government" in Chapter 7 and Section "Health Information Technology and Digital Health" in Chapter 4).

Telehealth goes beyond telemedicine to encompass some population health activities to keep patients healthy outside of an exam room (or Zoom screen). This may include remote monitoring from digital devices like blood pressure or glucose monitors. It may also mean getting a patient portal message from a medical assistant, asking you to book a mammogram online. These activities are relatively simple from a technologic point of view, and they align with our modern sense of improving health care quality—yet many clinics and health systems struggle to implement them. In some cases,

---

[c]State laws do exist barring practicing across state lines, including seeing your own doctor when you are in another state. These were temporarily waived during the pandemic but some are starting to be enforced again, limiting the use of telemedicine.

technology has outpaced the capabilities of the delivery system to effectively use it, even when they could be reimbursed for it. Although some institutions, like Ochsner Health in Louisiana, have demonstrated success with using remote monitoring,[56] for instance, these are still relatively rare examples to emulate rather than the norm.

Technology and telehealth have also blurred the lines between "care delivered in a clinic" and "care at home." Even though the *Ecology of Medical Care* didn't change much between 1961 and 2001, can we expect telemedicine to change this by 2041?

Home Health and Home-Based Care

People receive various types of medical care in their homes, potentially encompassing all 800 of our *Ecology* patients who experience symptoms. No one's counting if your mom comes over to bring you chicken soup when you have a cold, of course, but about 4.5 million adults receive home care services (otherwise known as "long-term services and supports" or LTSS).[57,d] Although quite a bit of advanced medical care can be delivered at home— including intravenous infusions—many people need much simpler help to stay well. About 20% of people over age 75 need nonprofessional help with activities like chores, shopping, cooking, and taking medications.[58] Yet those needs are often not met—for example, nearly half of older adults reporting difficulties with bathing and using the toilet had no equipment (such as grab bars) to help,[59] leaving them at high risk for falls and other bad outcomes.

The primary professionals who provide home care are home health aides and nurses, coming from about 12,000 agencies.[57] The primary *caregivers*, though, are nonprofessional and unpaid family members. Estimates indicate that 65 million Americans—the majority female and many of them older adults themselves—care for loved ones in the home with chronic conditions, disabilities, disease, or the frailties of old age.[60] The "average" U.S. caregiver is a 49-year-old woman who works outside the home then spends an additional 24 hours per week providing unpaid care to a parent for 4 years.[61]

Despite an aging population and those unmet needs, Medicare pays for in-home care under only very limited circumstances. Just over half of LTSS costs are paid for—if they're paid at all—by Medicaid instead. The payments, rules, and activities covered are complex and vary from state to state. Simple home care for those who need it—like meeting needs such as housing and food—may not be a "medical service" per se, but it is an essential prerequisite for the success of medical treatments. For instance, choosing the

---

[d] A large number of medically complex children also receive home care, though the CDC doesn't keep track of these numbers as they do for adults.

Median Annual Cost for Long-Term Care, 2015

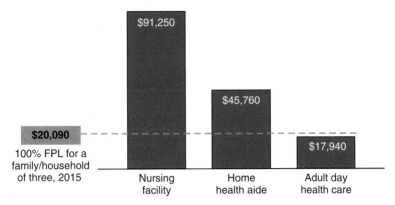

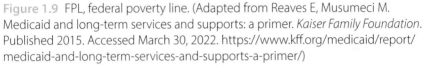

Figure 1.9 FPL, federal poverty line. (Adapted from Reaves E, Musumeci M. Medicaid and long-term services and supports: a primer. *Kaiser Family Foundation*. Published 2015. Accessed March 30, 2022. https://www.kff.org/medicaid/report/ medicaid-and-long-term-services-and-supports-a-primer/)

optimal medication regimen for heart failure is besides the point if a patient cannot manage their medications, get to the grocery store, or safely walk to the bathroom. It's also much cheaper to help people with these things in their own homes than to move them to nursing homes, as shown in Figure 1.9. In recognition of this, funding home care is a growing policy priority.[e]

One well-known subset of home care is called hospice, focused on care at the end of life (EOL).[f] Hospice programs shift emphasis to maximize quality of life rather than "quantity" of life for patients with terminal illnesses. Care is focused on providing comfort from their symptoms, including pain control, rather than attempting to cure the underlying cause. Fifty percent of Medicare beneficiaries who died in 2018 were under the care of a hospice program at the time of death.[62] For most patients, hospice care is associated with fewer days in the hospital and less Medicare spending (see Section "Complex Care Doesn't Come Cheap" in Chapter 3).[63]

All 1,000 People in the Ecology of Care

The Public Health System

Patients might not interface directly with the public health system, but it is the foundation of all care we receive, aiming to affect the entire 1,000 people

---

[e]In 2021, the American Rescue Plan increased federal matching payments to states that increased their LTSS.

[f]Hospice care is not exclusive to the home and can also be provided within a facility.

in our ecology of care. Public health touches our lives and wellness in ways we might not consider, such as in the workplace, in sanitation, in ensuring product safety and air quality. After all, although a doctor prescribes an inhaler if you have asthma, a pharmacist dispenses it, and a nurse teaches you to use it, who is going to recognize that you developed asthma because of poor air quality (poor air quality is the leading cause of chronic lung disease globally![64]) and ensure pollution is kept low to prevent disease?

In the United States, the public health system encompasses federal, state, and local (usually county) components (Table 1.2). Federal agencies do not deliver care but rather gather data and set policy—chances are you are quite familiar with the guidance of the CDC during the COVID-19 pandemic, for example (see Section "Federal Health Administration" in Chapter 6). State and local departments of health are a little more structurally complicated (ie, where they fall in the hierarchy of state governance), but they generally do similar work across states, including setting state policy as well as delivering

Table 1.2 Levels and Activities of the U.S. Public Health System

Federal 21 federal agencies including those you might naturally think of (CDC, FDA) and those you might not (EPA, Dept. of Agriculture)	■ Oversee the control of infection and chronic disease ■ Set standards and regulate food and product safety ■ Regulate environmental hazards ■ Support research ■ Evaluate new or rare diseases
State All 50 states have a public health agency; 29 are independent, whereas 21 are part of a bigger agency.	■ License health care workers ■ Run programs focused on public health topics such as maternal health, tobacco control, and environmental health ■ Track disease and gather statistics ■ Maintain immunization registries ■ Organize response to public health emergencies
Local 2,459 local health departments	■ Regulate and license businesses such as restaurants ■ Inspect potential environmental hazards ■ Respond to foodborne illness reports ■ Run immunization and screening programs ■ Educate and do outreach for public health topics

EPA, U.S. Environmental Protection Agency.
Source: Adapted from M Wallace, JM Sharfstein. The patchwork U.S. public health system. *N Engl J Med.* 2022;386:1-4. doi:10.1056/NEJMp2104881

some care, such as vaccines, sexually transmitted infection testing and treatment, and tuberculosis care.

Another way public health touches care is through partnerships and community health needs assessments. These are annual surveys of exactly what they sound like. You can look one up in your own community.

The "Safety Net"

Technically, the American health care safety net is defined as "providers that organize and deliver a significant level of health care and other needed services to uninsured, Medicaid, and other vulnerable patients." Metaphorically, though, that "net" is more like hanging a moth-eaten patchwork quilt under a tightrope walker.

Delivery of care in the safety net is often managed by the government. Examples of the safety net discussed in this chapter include CHCs/FQHCs, critical access hospitals, and the public health system. Medicaid, discussed in Chapter 2, is part of the safety net because it insures the most vulnerable. (Even EDs, mandated by law to evaluate anyone regardless of ability to pay, are an element of the safety net.) In many cases, the responsibility for uninsured and low-income patients falls on a county, but how this looks varies. Some counties operate clinics and a hospital directly through their Department of Public Health, whereas others pay for the care of the underserved through the private delivery system, such as not-for-profit and academic hospitals.

Nongovernment-run hospitals are also a component of the safety net. In 2018, community hospitals reported $40 billion in charity care and bad debt.[65] Recognizing that this uncompensated care tends to cluster in certain community hospitals that serve a higher number of uninsured and Medicaid patients, Medicaid has made disproportionate share hospital (DSH) payments since the 1980s. The ACA reduced DSH payments, the idea being that because more people would be insured, hospitals wouldn't have to provide as much uncompensated care, but reductions have mostly been deferred. In 2019, hospitals received $19.7 billion in DSH payments.[66] Rural, teaching, children's, and not-for-profit hospitals are more likely to receive these payments.[65]

Low-income, uninsured, Medicaid, and vulnerable populations don't just need medical care. An important element of the safety net is addressing SDoH, such as access to food, housing, employment opportunities, and transportation. Depending on where you live, these resources may be fairly robust, or they may be practically nonexistent; in either case, patients may not access resources simply because they don't know what is available to them. Imagine that tightrope walker falling through a hole in the patchwork quilt. If only a spectator had shouted "Lean a little to the left!" they could have been caught.

We rely heavily on medical social workers (MSWs; page 228) to be that voice, but as MSWs do not get reimbursed by insurance for their services, many systems do not employ enough of them despite their importance to team-based care.

Population Health and Delivery Innovations

Although traditionally the realm of public health, activities that affect the health of all 1,000 people are increasingly being taken on by medical providers and delivery organizations, such as large hospital networks, primary care clinics, and even insurance companies themselves. This is similar in principle to public health but different in scope, because it only applies to the people who seek care at these organizations (ie, the organization's "population"). Rather than public health, which is run by the government to serve all people living in a place (ie, "the public"), we call this "population health."

Population health has no universally accepted definition, but the American Association of Medical Colleges (AAMC) considers it "a systematic approach to ensuring that all members of a defined population receive appropriate preventive, chronic, and transitional care."[67] This involves thinking beyond the patients scheduled on a given day, to ask instead "what are the total health outcomes for our patients over time, even those who aren't coming in, and how can I improve those outcomes" even if the way to improve them isn't with a doctor's appointment.

Some Common Population Health Interventions

- **Ensuring Quick Access to Care:** Sometimes this means keeping a clinic open during evenings and weekends, an after-hours call line, or "holding" slots for last-minute appointments.
- **Identifying and Focusing on High-Risk, High-Needs Patients:** This might be through tracking ED visits or by types of medical problems. It also might mean investing in nonmedical interventions like transportation and housing.[g]
- **Building Larger Medical Teams Beyond Physicians:** These may include nurses, social workers, care coaches, dietitians, community health workers, pharmacists, and more. It also involves coordinating that care among independent groups, and focusing on directing services toward high-value providers.

---

[g]Like UnitedHealth, which had invested $500 million in housing as of 2020. (https://www.forbes.com/sites/brucejapsen/2020/06/04/unitedhealth-group-boosts-housing-investments-to-500m-to-address-social-determinants/?sh=44d570b32815)

- **Proactive Patient Outreach Rather Than Waiting for Patients to Come In:** This requires both knowing how often different patients *should* come in, as well as tracking when they do.
- **Greater Focus on Transitions of Care:** This means tracking when patients get admitted and discharged, ensuring nothing slips through the cracks (see Section "Transitions in Care" in Chapter 4), and that patients get timely access to next steps with their outpatient clinicians.

One population health delivery innovation that's gotten a lot of attention is called "hotspotting." Hotspotting means focusing on high-needs, high-cost patients (see Section "How Is That Spending Distributed Through the Population?" in Chapter 3) and bringing medical care to the patients—for instance, on the streets—rather than bringing the patients to a medical care facility.[68,h] Although there has since been a lot of similar work focused on interventions for the highest cost patients, this was called into question when a randomized controlled trial of hotspotting by the Camden Coalition was published in 2020 and showed no ongoing reduction in hospital readmissions for patients.[69] As with many areas of health care, even a great idea might not generate the outcomes hoped for.

Population health management is also a strategy used to save money in the long run by investing in outpatient care to prevent costly inpatient and post-acute care. However, systems need help with up-front costs of building new programs. The ACA created the CMMI or CMS Innovation Center, which functions to test nontraditional payment and delivery models around the nation (see Section "Paying for Innovation: CMS Innovation Center" in Chapter 6, Section "APMs and Value-Based Payment" in Chapter 3). These types of alternative payment models (APMs) offer bonuses or penalties to incentivize certain types of high-quality care: CMMI has programs focused on dialysis, joint surgery, primary care, and oncology care, among many others. However, it's important to remember that APMs focus not just on delivering care differently but delivering it differently *at lower total cost.* This means that these programs also rely on:

- Documenting patient conditions to adjust spending based on medical risk
- Access to EHR and insurance data
- Encouraging patients to receive care from the most efficient health care providers and facilities (often focused on reducing ER visits and hospitalizations)

---

[h]Dr. Brenner won a MacArthur Genius grant in 2013 for his hotspotting work with the Camden Coalition.

It is difficult to draw any conclusions about the overall impact these delivery innovations have on health care cost, quality, and access—so far, just like with hotspotting, it's been a mixed bag.[70] CMMI coordinates many of the largest APM programs in the United States and reports that although most have demonstrated improved quality, the majority have lost money, with several on pace to lose billions of dollars (see Section "Paying for Innovation: CMS Innovation Center" in Chapter 6).[71]

Issues in Care Delivery

Now that we've gone over the basics, let's address a few of the problems and complexities in care delivery that you are likely to hear about.

Access

In this chapter, we've given you an idea of the scope of how and where medical care is delivered. It's one thing for hospitals and clinics to be there—but what about getting patients into them? Patients' ability to actually get appointments for their care is a major issue for almost all clinicians and health systems.

You may have heard about long wait times in other countries. You may have even waited a long time for an appointment yourself. Generally, we can think about access in three domains: first, finding a clinician who takes your insurance; second, scheduling a timely appointment; and third, physically getting to the appointment.

First, finding a clinician who takes your insurance. Although this can be a struggle for anyone, it is perhaps most so for patients on Medicaid—and even harder for patients without any insurance at all (see Section "Medicaid and CHIP" in Chapter 2). Based on polling of physicians, only 68% of family doctors said they would take a new patient with Medicaid, compared to a patient on Medicare or private insurance (both 90%).[72] (Notably, based on secret shopper calls, that 68% rate dropped to 53%.)[73] It is much worse if you need mental health care: only 35% of psychiatrists say they would accept a patient on Medicaid.[72]

Second, scheduling a timely appointment. As with many issues in U.S. health care, there is a huge amount of variation here, depending on geography, insurance status, and type of medical center. As you read the averages, it's important to note both the wide variation as well as the lack of transparency. The average wait to see a new family doctor in a major city is 29 days, ranging from 8 days in Minneapolis to 109 days in Boston. To see an orthopedic surgeon, that wait is an average of 11 days, ranging from 1 day in many cities to 180 days in Detroit. Wait times get even longer in smaller cities, where a new patient might wait 32 days to see a cardiologist or 35 days to see a dermatologist.[73]

You may have read in 2014 about the VA wait times scandal (in short, because the Arizona VA wasn't meeting its goal of a 14-day wait or less for appointments, they kept a secret wait list to falsify metrics).[74] Despite this scandal, research found that, actually, overall VA wait times for clinic visits were comparable to the private sector, and, when updated in 2017, VA clinics were actually faster (17 days) on average than the private sector (29 days).[75]

Finally, part of access is managing to arrive at your appointment. This is an issue for those who have trouble taking off work (particularly if they don't have sick leave), who live far from where they can get care, and who might not have access to a car.[i] And although telehealth might solve some of those problems, it creates new ones, limiting health care access for those without technology and internet capabilities.

When the ACA increased the number of people with insurance, there were fears that suddenly access would worsen, as more and more people tried to get appointments with the same number of physicians. Luckily, studies have largely found that, overall, wait times remained stable.[76]

Some behaviors and trends in other areas of delivery and policy are rooted in problems of access. For instance, there is a lot of attention on patients who go to the ED for simple, nonemergency problems. But for many people, the ED might be the only way to access care when they need it—a place that's always open and won't turn them away for lack of payment. On the other end of the spectrum, the growth in concierge and on-demand telehealth appointments reflects the market meeting the demand of patients who want improved access and are willing to pay for it.

The ability to access care in a timely fashion is of utmost importance to the patients receiving that care; thus, it is a major concern for any clinic or hospital.

Rural–Urban Divide

Just because medical care is available doesn't mean everyone can access it, or that they can access it equally. Inequities in care and outcomes exist along many lines—such as ethnicity, language, and class—but let's look at one in particular: the rural–urban divide.

Rural populations have the highest mortality rate.[77] They are more likely to be uninsured and to stay uninsured for longer.[78] They are less likely to see dentists[79] and less likely to receive flu shots.[80] They have higher rates of

---

[i]A study looking at transportation benefits in an APM found that while this program wasn't cost-saving in terms of health expenditures, it did ease patient financial burden significantly. Berkowitz SA, Ricks KB, Wang J, Parker M, Rimal R, DeWalt DA. Evaluating a nonemergency medical transportation benefit for accountable care organization members. *Health Aff (Millwood)*. 2022;41(3): 406-413. doi:10.1377/hlthaff.2021.00449

chronic disease like emphysema and heart disease and are more likely to die from it.[77,81] They are less likely to be screened for colorectal cancer,[82] and, if diagnosed, they have far fewer specialists available, like gastroenterologists or radiation oncologists, to receive treatment from.[83] Rural veterans are more likely to die by suicide.[84] Rural children are more likely to have mental, behavioral, and development disorders.[85] Rural stroke victims are less likely to receive a medication that can reverse a stroke.[86]

So if you live in a rural area, not only are you less likely to be able to get somewhere you can receive medical treatment, but you might have worse health outcomes even when you do. And the disparity only seems to worsen over time. Most notably, rural hospitals and nursing homes are closing—a trend accelerated by the COVID-19 pandemic—meaning people have to travel farther for care or to see their loved ones in facilities.[87,88]

Because of the risks to those who live in rural areas, the government sometimes steps in to ensure delivery where the market might not. One example of this is critical access hospitals (CAHs; Figure 1.10). CAHs are small (<25 beds), generally must be at least 35 miles from any other hospital, and must have 24/7 emergency services. These hospitals get extra funding through both Medicare and Medicaid to help prevent closures that would leave rural communities without any hospitals at all. The government supports a patchwork of other programs[89] intended to increase resources for rural health.

Another example of government-supported rural access is the IHS, which is a federal agency serving about 2.5 million Native Americans,[90] a population that is disproportionately rural and experiences significant health disparities. The IHS delivers care but is not itself an insurance benefit[90] (in contrast to the Veterans Health Administration or TRICARE; see Chapter 2).

Nurse Staffing

Although some health care delivery topics can seem hopelessly complex, others are fairly intuitive; for example, it's more difficult for a nurse to take care of 10 patients at the same time than to take care of 4 patients. Nurse staffing, or the ratio of how many patients a nurse is supposed to care for, is also impacted by the educational level of the nursing and ancillary staff as well as by how sick the patients are (eg, ICU patients require more nursing attention).

Dozens of studies have shown the dramatic impact that nurse staffing has on a number of outcomes, including[91]:

■ Reduced patient mortality, readmissions, failure to rescue, medication errors, length of stay, falls, pressure ulcers, hospital-acquired infections
■ Increased patient satisfaction

Map of 5,250 Acute Care and Critical Access Hospitals

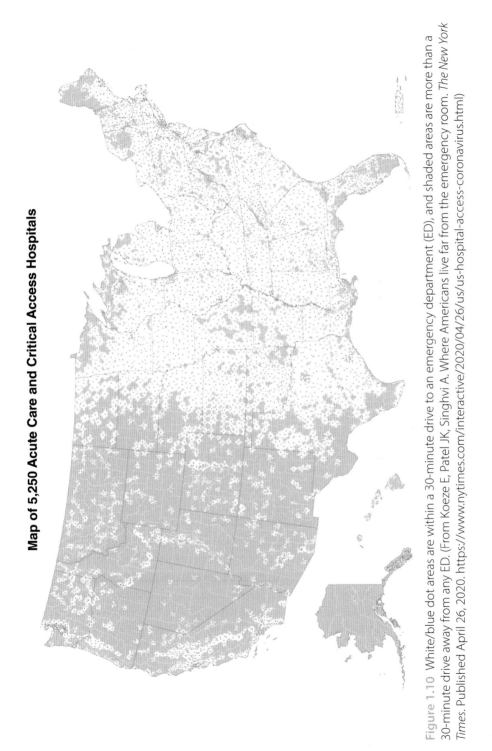

Figure 1.10 White/blue dot areas are within a 30-minute drive to an emergency department (ED), and shaded areas are more than a 30-minute drive away from any ED. (From Koeze E, Patel JK, Singhvi A. Where Americans live far from the emergency room. *The New York Times*. Published April 26, 2020. https://www.nytimes.com/interactive/2020/04/26/us/us-hospital-access-coronavirus.html)

■ Increased job satisfaction among nurses, with reduced burnout and staff turnover

Recognizing the importance of nurse staffing, several states have passed legislation to ensure adequate nurse staffing at hospitals. The oldest and most studied policy was passed in California in 2004, which limits nurses to no more than five general medical/surgical patients, or two ICU patients.[92] The policy has been effective in improving nursing job satisfaction and reducing occupational injuries but, surprisingly, studies have not found any substantial improvement in patient outcomes.[93]

Although nurse staffing is well-recognized as critical to patient care, hospitals and SNFs across the country still struggle to adequately staff their hospital beds for a number of reasons, including variability in patient volume and acuity, local shortages in available nurses, and tight hospital budgets (though some studies show increasing nursing staff generates positive financial return on the extra expense).[94] It's worth mentioning that paying registered nurses represents 25% of hospital budgets.[95]

All of these factors were pushed to the forefront simultaneously during the COVID-19 pandemic. Over and over, in different areas of the country, rising cases led to overfilled hospitals, yet restrictions on the supply of nurses (because of exposures and quarantine, or simply an inability to maintain staff) meant some hospitals didn't have enough nurses to use all of their open beds. Remaining nurses were often required to take on a larger load of sicker patients.

Aside from the chronic problem of nurse staffing ratios, hiring and retaining nurses at all is becoming a problem. In a 2021 poll of nurses, about half said they were likely or extremely likely to leave bedside nursing within the next 2 years.[96] Some nurses aren't leaving the profession altogether, but are quitting to become travel nurses (travel nurses work temporary positions, in which they can make more money than being hired full-time).[97] Although the Bureau of Labor Statistics currently projects that job growth for nurses will remain at about the average for all occupations, some worry that this might change, as concerns over staffing ratios, salary, and burnout encourage more nurses to leave the workforce. As such, many nursing organizations, such as the American Association of Colleges of Nursing, lobby for legislation to help fund initiatives to increase and support the nursing workforce.[98]

Primary Care Problems

Primary care stands out from the rest of our *Ecology of Medical Care*, bridging the gap between medical care for specialized acute illnesses and health promotion for the whole person. Primary care provides the first—and oftentimes only—step of medical evaluation and treatment, by a physician, nurse practitioner, or physician assistant. In conjunction with a health team, these clinicians are responsible for diagnosing and addressing a wide range of medical problems while maintaining a long-term relationship with patients.

Primary care delivers the bulk of care, yet only 5% to 7% of all health spending goes to primary care.[99] Only one-third of practicing physicians are in primary care currently, and fewer than one-fourth of current medical graduates plan to go into it in the future.[100] This proportion of primary care clinicians per population is lower than any other comparable country—the Organisation for Economic Co-operation and Development (OECD) lists the density of generalists per 1,000 population as 0.3 in the United States, 0.76 in the United Kingdom, 1.01 in Germany, 1.4 in France, and 1.7 in Australia.[101] In other words, in the United States, there's one generalist for every 3,300 people; in Australia, there's one for every 588 people.

A large workload falls on these clinicians' shoulders. Duke University researchers estimate that, given the typical patient load and the current guidelines for care, a primary care provider (PCP) should be spending 7.4 hours per day on preventive care, 10.6 hours on managing chronic diseases,[25] and 4.6 hours on handling acute illness[26]—totaling 22.6 hours a day.[4] Writing notes to document visits adds another hour,[102] and increasing requirements to report and meet quality metrics (such as for Medicare's Quality Payment Program or APMs) may further require time spent away from patients themselves (see Section "EHRs and Burnout" in Chapter 4). Finally, the increase in uncompensated digital work (such as messages from patients) during the pandemic has only increased the workload.[103] (Perhaps surprisingly, only 46% of PCPs—comparable to other specialties—report burnout.[104])

Why does the strain on primary care matter? The Institute of Medicine (IOM) lists five ways in which primary care is valuable to society:

1. It provides a place to which patients can bring a wide range of health problems for appropriate attention—a place in which patients can expect, in most instances, that their problems will be resolved without referral.

2. It guides patients through the health system, including appropriate referrals for services from other health professionals.

3. It facilitates an ongoing relationship between patients and clinicians and fosters participation by patients in decision-making about their health and their own care.

4. It provides opportunities for disease prevention and health promotion as well as early detection of problems.

5. It helps build bridges between personal health care services and patients' families and communities that can assist in meeting the health needs of the patient.[105]

Some wish to fix primary care's problems by paying PCPs more, and it's true that PCPs receive lower payment relative to specialists, earning only 61% of what specialists make[106] (see Section "Setting Payments to Physicians, Part 1: the RUC" in Chapter 6). But ensuring robust primary care as a field that people want to work in will require more than money: it will take a coordinated effort to change payment systems (such as Section "Alternative Payment Models and Value-Based Payment" in Chapter 3), reduce documentation burden (such as the changes in Medicare billing requirements in 2021), streamline inefficiencies (such as aligning billing workflows between insurance plans and reducing paperwork), and build strong teams (with nonclinician staff).

Many think our current FFS reimbursement system simply cannot adequately account for and reward the work of a PCP and primary care clinic, and some APMs employ different methods of reimbursement to do so. One such well-known model is the Patient-Centered Medical Home, which has been established in over 10,000 practices.[107] Yet most of the models are being adopted slowly, still rely on FFS payments, and are quite complex to figure out, meaning that the models favor consolidation over independent practices (PCPs would generally rather see patients than figure out obscure new reimbursement rules). To help with such problems, in 2021, primary care experts called for the creation of a government body that can create and implement a coordinated primary care strategy nationwide.[108]

References

1. Green LA, Fryer GE Jr, Yawn BP, Lanier D, Dovey SM. The ecology of medical care revisited. *N Engl J Med*. 2001;344(26):2021-2025. doi:10.1056/NEJM200106283442611
2. White KL, Williams TF, Greenberg BG. The ecology of medical care. *N Engl J Med*. 1961;265:885-892.
3. National Association of State Emergency Medical Services Officials. 2020 national emergency medical services assessment. Published May 27, 2020. https://nasemso.org/wp-content/uploads/2020-National-EMS-Assessment_Reduced-File-Size.pdf
4. Chhabra KR, McGuire K, Sheetz KH, Scott JW, Nuliyalu U, Ryan AM. Most patients undergoing ground and air ambulance transportation receive sizable out-of-network bills. *Health Aff (Millwood)*. 2020;39(5):777-782. doi:10.1377/hlthaff.2019.01484
5. Centers for Disease Control and Prevention. Emergency department visits. Accessed March 25, 2022. https://www.cdc.gov/nchs/fastats/emergency-department.htm
6. Agency for Healthcare Research and Quality. MEPS HC-197E: 2017 emergency room visits. Published June, 2019. https://meps.ahrq.gov/data_stats/download_data/pufs/h197e/h197edoc.pdf
7. Cairns C, Ashman J, Kang K. Emergency department visit rates by selected characteristics: United States, 2018. *Centers for Disease Control and Prevention*. Published March, 2021. https://www.cdc.gov/nchs/products/databriefs/db401.htm
8. Hooker EA, Mallow PJ, Oglesby MM. Characteristics and trends of emergency department visits in the United States (2010-2014). *J Emerg Med*. 2019;56(3):344-351. doi:10.1016/j.jemermed.2018.12.025

9. Bellolio MF, Heien HC, Sangaralingham LR, et al. Increased computed tomography utilization in the emergency department and its association with hospital admission. *West J Emerg Med*. 2017;18(5):835-845. doi:10.5811/westjem.2017.5.34152

10. Bureau of Labor Statistics, U.S. Department of Labor, Number of hospitals and hospital employment in each state in 2019. *The Economics Daily*. Accessed July 2, 2022. https://www.bls.gov/opub/ted/2020/number-of-hospitals-and-hospital-employment-in-each-state-in-2019.htm

11. American Hospital Association. Fast facts on U.S. hospitals, 2022. Published January, 2022. https://www.aha.org/statistics/fast-facts-us-hospitals

12. Mitchell M. Certificate-of-need laws: how they affect healthcare access, quality, and cost. Published May 21, 2021. https://www.mercatus.org/Certificate-of-Need-Laws-How-They-Affect-Healthcare-Access-Quality-and-Cost

13. Erickson A. States are suspending certificate of need laws in the wake of COVID-19 but the damage might already be done. *Pacific Legal Foundation*. Published January 11, 2021. https://pacificlegal.org/certificate-of-need-laws-covid-19/

14. Military Health System. MHS health facilities. Published August 5, 2021. https://www.health.mil/I-Am-A/Media/Media-Center/MHS-Health-Facilities

15. Indian Health Service. *IHS profile*. Published August, 2020. https://www.ihs.gov/newsroom/factsheets/ihsprofile/

16. Veterans Health Administration. *About VHA*. Published May 24, 2022. https://www.va.gov/health/aboutVHA.asp

17. PEW. Prison health care costs and quality. Published October 18, 2017. https://www.pewtrusts.org/en/research-and-analysis/reports/2017/10/prison-health-care-costs-and-quality

18. American Hospital Association. Teaching hospitals. https://www.aha.org/advocacy/teaching-hospitals

19. Heath S. Does hospital religious affiliation impact patient access to care? *Patient Engagement HIT*. Published January 2, 2020. https://patientengagementhit.com/news/does-hospital-religious-affiliation-impact-patient-access-to-care

20. Casimir G. Why children's hospitals are unique and so essential. *Front Pediatr*. 2019;7:305. doi:10.3389/fped.2019.00305

21. HCA Healthcare. HCA healthcare fact sheet. Published June 30, 2019. https://hcahealthcare.com/util/forms/press-kit/HCA-presskit-fact-sheet-a.pdf

22. King R. Hospital groups demand CMS halt expansion of certain physician-owned hospitals in payment rule. *Fierce Healthcare*. Published October 6, 2020. https://www.fiercehealthcare.com/hospitals/hospital-groups-demand-cms-halt-expansion-certain-doc-owned-hospitals-payment-rule

23. Inglehart JK. The emergence of physician-owned specialty hospitals. *N Engl J Med*. 2005;352(1):78-84.

24. HCUP Fast Stats. Healthcare Cost and Utilization Project (HCUP). *Agency for Healthcare Research and Quality*. April, 2021. www.houp-us.ahrq.gov/faststats/national/inpatient-commondiagnoses.jsp

25. Poon SJ, Wallis CJD, Lai P, Podczerwinski L, Buntin MB. Medicare two-midnight rule accelerated shift to observation stays. *Health Aff (Millwood)*. 2021;40(11):1688-1696. doi:10.1377/hlthaff.2021.00094

26. Tian W. An all-payer view of hospital discharge to postacute care, 2013. HCUP Statistical Brief #205. *Agency for Healthcare Research and Quality*. May, 2016. http://www.hcup-us.ahrq.gov/reports/statbriefs/sb205-Hospital-Discharge-Postacute-Care.pdf

27. American Hospital Association. Fact sheet: post-acute care. Published July, 2019. https://www.aha.org/system/files/media/file/2019/07/fact-sheet-post-acute-care-0719.pdf

28. Medicare Payment Advisory Commission. March 2022 Report to the Congress: Chapter 10 Long term care hospital services (p. 343). Published March, 2022. https://www.medpac.gov/wp-content/uploads/2022/03/Mar22_MedPAC_ReportToCongress_Ch10_SEC.pdf

29. Mechanic R. Post-acute care—the next frontier for controlling Medicare spending. *N Engl J Med*. 2014;370(8):692-694. doi:10.1056/NEJMp1315607

30. Gandhi A, Yu H, Grabowski DC. High nursing staff turnover in nursing homes offers important quality information. *Health Aff (Millwood)*. 2021;40(3):384-391. doi:10.1377/hlthaff.2020.00957

31. Flynn M. Median skilled nursing margin breaks even, but 'Long-Term Financial Viability is Uncertain.' *Skilled Nursing News*. Published January 8, 2020. https://skillednursingnews.com/2020/01/median-skilled-nursing-margin-breaks-even-but-long-term-financial-viability-is-uncertain/

32. Rui P, Okeyode T. National ambulatory medical care survey: 2016 national summary tables. https://www.cdc.gov/nchs/data/ahcd/namcs_summary/2016_namcs_web_tables.pdf

33. Ashman JJ, Rui P, Okeyode T. Characteristics of office-based physician visits, 2016. NCHS Data Brief, no 331. National Center for Health Statistics. 2019. https://www.cdc.gov/nchs/products/databriefs/db331.htm

34. Nursing Center. U.S. nurses in 2020: who we are and where we work. 2020. https://www.nursingcenter.com/nursingcenter_redesign/media/nursingcenter/Infographics/U-S-Nurses-2020.png

35. National Association of Community Health Centers. America's health centers: 2021 snapshot. Published August, 2021. https://www.nachc.org/research-and-data/research-fact-sheets-and-infographics/americas-health-centers-2021-snapshot/

36. Definitive Healthcare. How many federally qualified health centers are there? https://blog.definitivehc.com/how-many-fqhcs-are-there

37. Velan M. Booming urgent care industry fills the gaps in patient care. *Urgent Care Association*. Published February 7, 2019. https://www.ucaoa.org/About-UCA/Industry-News/ArtMID/10309/ArticleID/877/Booming-Urgent-Care-Industry-Filling-the-Gaps-in-Patient-Care

38. Butler S, Barkley E, MacGibbon A, et al. Urgent care shifts to testing and immunization during the pandemic. *Epic Research*. Published December 7, 2021. https://epicresearch.org/articles/urgent-care-shifts-to-testing-and-immunization-during-the-pandemic

39. CVS Pharmacy. About us: history. https://www.cvs.com/minuteclinic/visit/about-us/history

40. Steiner CA, Karaca Z, Moore BJ, Imshaug MC, Pickens G. Surgeries in hospital-based ambulatory surgery and hospital inpatient settings, 2014. HCUP Statistical Brief #223. *Agency for Healthcare Research and Quality*. May 2017. www.hcup-us.ahrq.gov/reports/statbriefs/sb223-Ambulatory-Inpatient-Surgeries-2014.pdf

41. Definitive Healthcare. How many ambulatory surgery centers are in the U.S.? https://www.definitivehc.com/blog/how-many-ascs-are-in-the-us

42. Definitive Healthcare. Top 10 outpatient procedures at surgery centers and hospitals. Updated May 22, 2019. https://www.definitivehc.com/blog/top-10-outpatient-procedures-at-ascs-and-hospitals

43. Ambulatory Surgery Center Association. ASCs: a positive trend in health care. *Advancing Surgical Care*. https://www.ascassociation.org/advancingsurgicalcare/aboutascs/industryoverview/apositivetrendinhealthcare

44. Centers for Disease Control and Prevention. Chronic kidney disease surveillance system—United States. https://nccd.cdc.gov/ckd/

45. Healthcare Appraisers. 2020 outlook: dialysis clinics and ESRD. Published May 6, 2020. https://healthcareappraisers.com/2020-outlook-dialysis-clinics-and-esrd/

46. Pew Research Center. Vast majority of Americans say benefits of childhood vaccines outweigh risks. Published February 2, 2017. https://www.pewresearch.org/science/2017/02/02/vast-majority-of-americans-say-benefits-of-childhood-vaccines-outweigh-risks/

47. Freed M, Ochieng N, Sroczynski N, et al. Medicare and dental coverage: a closer look. *Kaiser Family Foundation*. Published July 28, 2021. https://www.kff.org/medicare/issue-brief/medicare-and-dental-coverage-a-closer-look/

48. National Institutes of Health. Americans spent $30.2 billion out-of-pocket on complementary health approaches. Published June 22, 2016. https://www.nih.gov/news-events/americans-spent-302-billion-out-pocket-complementary-health-approaches

49. Hoffman J. CVS, Walgreens and Walmart fueled opioid crisis, jury finds. *New York Times*. Published November 23, 2021. https://www.nytimes.com/2021/11/23/health/walmart-cvs-opioid-lawsuit-verdict.html

50. Qato DM, Zenk S, Wilder J, Harrington R, Gaskin D, Alexander GC. The availability of pharmacies in the United States: 2007-2015. *PLoS One*. 2017;12(8):e0183172. doi:10.1371/journal.pone.0183172

51. Hawryluk M. The last drugstore: rural America is losing its pharmacies. *Washington Post*. Published November 10, 2021. https://www.washingtonpost.com/business/2021/11/10/drugstore-shortage-rural-america/?utm_source=feedly&utm_medium=referral&utm_campaign=wp_homepage

52. Sierra S, Feingold L, Manthey G. 'A Huge Disparity': San Francisco, Oakland neighborhoods struggle with pharmacy deserts. *ABC 7 News*. Published January 15, 2021. https://abc7news.com/pharmacy-deserts-oakland-san-francisco-covid-19-vaccine/9696783/

53. Seeley E, Singh S. Competition, consolidation, and evolution in the pharmacy market: implications for efforts to contain drug prices and spending. *Commonwealth Fund*. doi:10.26099/exwh-r479

54. Bosworth A, Ruhter J, Samson LW, et al. Medicare beneficiary use of telehealth visits: early data from the start of COVID-19 pandemic. Office of the Assistant Secretary for Planning and Evaluation, U.S. Department of Health and Human Services. Published July 28, 2020. https://aspe.hhs.gov/reports/medicare-beneficiary-use-telehealth-visits-early-data-start-covid-19-pandemic

55. Demeke HB, Merali S, Marks S, et al. Trends in use of telehealth among health centers during the COVID-19 pandemic—United States, June 26-November 6, 2020. *MMWR Morb Mortal Wkly Rep*. 2021;70:240-244. doi:10.15585/mmwr.mm7007a3

56. American Medical Association. Ochsner health—hypertension digital medicine program. Published May 2021. https://www.ama-assn.org/system/files/2021-05/case-study-ochsner-health-hypertension-digital-medicine-program.pdf

57. Harris-Kojetin L, Sengupta M, Lendon JP, Rome V, Valverde R, Caffrey C. Long-term care providers and services users in the United States, 2015-2016. National Center for Health Statistics. *Vital Health Stat*. 2019;3(43).

58. Lucas JW, Benson V. Tables of summary health statistics for the U.S. population: 2018 national health interview survey. National Center for Health Statistics. 2019. https://www.cdc.gov/nchs/nhis/SHS/tables.htm.

59. Lam K, Shi Y, Boscardin J, Covinsky KE. Unmet need for equipment to help with bathing and toileting among older US adults. *JAMA Intern Med.* 2021;181(5):662-670. doi:10.1001/jamainternmed.2021.0204

60. American Psychological Association. Who are family caregivers? 2011. https://www.apa.org/pi/about/publications/caregivers/faq/statistics

61. Family Caregiver Alliance. Caregiver statistics: demographics. 2016. https://www.caregiver.org/resource/caregiver-statistics-demographics/

62. *Hospice Facts and Figures.* National Hospice and Palliative Care Organization; 2020. www.nhpco.org/factsfigures

63. Zuckerman RB, Stearns SC, Sheingold SH. Hospice use, hospitalization, and Medicare spending at the end of life. *J Gerontol B Psychol Sci Soc Sci.* 2016;71(3):569-580. doi:10.1093/geronb/gbv109

64. GBD Chronic Respiratory Disease Collaborators. Prevalence and attributable health burden of chronic respiratory diseases, 1990-2017: a systematic analysis for the Global Burden of Disease Study 2017. *Lancet Respir Med.* 2020;8(6):585-596. doi:10.1016/S2213-2600(20)30105-3

65. Medicaid and CHIP Payment and Access Commission. Annual analysis of disproportionate share hospital allotments to states (p. 150). Published March, 2021. https://www.macpac.gov/wp-content/uploads/2021/03/Chapter-5-Annual-Analysis-of-Disproportionate-Share-Hospital-Allotments-to-States.pdf

66. Medicaid and CHIP Payment and Access Commission. Disproportionate share hospital payments. https://www.macpac.gov/subtopic/disproportionate-share-hospital-payments/

67. Bodenheimer T, Syer S, Fair M, Shipman S. Teaching residents population health management. *American Association of Medical Colleges.* Published November, 2019. https://store.aamc.org/teaching-residents-population-health-management.html

68. Gawande A. The hot spotters: can we lower medical costs by giving the neediest patients better care? *The New Yorker.* Published January 16, 2011. https://www.newyorker.com/magazine/2011/01/24/the-hot-spotters

69. Finkelstein A, Zhou A, Taubman S, Doyle J. Health care hotspotting—a randomized, controlled trial. *N Engl J Med.* 2020;382(2):152-162. doi:10.1056/NEJMsa1906848

70. Mendelson A, Kondo K, Damberg C, et al. The effects of pay-for-performance programs on health, health care use, and processes of care: a systematic review. *Ann Intern Med.* 2017;166(5):341-353. doi:10.7326/M16-1881

71. Smith B. CMS innovation center at 10 years—progress and lessons learned. *N Engl J Med.* 2021;384(8):759-764. doi:10.1056/NEJMsb2031138

72. Holgash K, Heberlein M. Physician acceptance of new Medicaid patients. Medicaid and CHIP Payment and Access Commission. Published January 24, 2019. https://www.macpac.gov/wp-content/uploads/2019/01/Physician-Acceptance-of-New-Medicaid-Patients.pdf

73. Merritt Hawkins. 2017 survey of physician appointment wait times and Medicare and Medicaid acceptance rates. https://www.merritthawkins.com/uploadedFiles/MerrittHawkins/Content/Pdf/mha2017waittimesurveyPDF.pdf

74. Lopez G. The VA scandal of 2014, explained. *Vox.* Updated May 13, 2015. https://www.vox.com/2014/9/26/18080592/va-scandal-explained

75. Penn M, Bhatnagar S, Kuy S, et al. Comparison of wait times for new patients between the private sector and United States Department of Veterans Affairs Medical Centers. *JAMA Netw Open.* 2019;2(1):e187096. doi:10.1001/jamanetworkopen.2018.7096

76. Mazurenko O, Balio CP, Agarwal R, Carroll AE, Menachemi N. The effects of Medicaid expansion under the ACA: a systematic review. *Health Aff (Millwood).* 2018;37(6):944-950. doi:10.1377/hlthaff.2017.1491

77. Cross SH, Mehra MR, Bhatt DL, et al. Rural-urban differences in cardiovascular mortality in the US, 1999-2017. *JAMA.* 2020;323(18):1852-1854. doi:10.1001/jama.2020.2047

78. Georgetown University. Health Policy Institute. Rural and urban health. https://hpi .georgetown.edu/rural/

79. Rural Health Information Hub. Oral health in rural communities. Accessed March 22, 2019. https://www.ruralhealthinfo.org/topics/oral-health

80. Martino, SC, Elliott, MN, Dembosky JW, et al. *Rural-Urban Disparities in Health Care in Medicare.* CMS Office of Minority Health; 2020.

81. Iyer AS, Cross SH, Dransfield MT, Warraich HJ. Urban-rural disparities in deaths from chronic lower respiratory disease in the United States. *Am J Respir Crit Care Med.* 2021;203(6):769-772. doi:10.1164/rccm.202008-3375LE

82. Office of Disease Prevention and Health Promotion. Health People 2020: Disparities overview by geographic location, C16: adults receiving colorectal cancer screening based on the most recent guidelines (age-adjusted, percent, 50-75 years). Department of Health and Human Services; 2020.

83. Aboagye JK, Kaiser HE, Hayanga AJ. Rural-urban differences in access to specialist providers of colorectal cancer care in the United States: a physician workforce issue. *JAMA Surg.* 2014;149(6):537-543. doi:10.1001/jamasurg.2013.5062

84. Shiner B, Peltzman T, Cornelius, SL, et al. Recent trends in the rural–urban suicide disparity among veterans using VA health care. *J Behav Med.* 2021;44:492-506. doi:10.1007/s10865-020-00176-9

85. Kelleher KJ, Gardner W. Out of sight, out of mind—behavioral and developmental care for rural children. *N Engl J Med.* 2017;376(14):1301-1303. doi:10.1056/NEJMp1700713

86. Gonzales S, Mullen MT, Skolarus L, Thibault DP, Udoeyo U, Willis AW. Progressive rural–urban disparity in acute stroke care. *Neurology.* 2017;88(5):441-448. doi:10.1212/WNL.0000000000003562

87. United States Government Accountability Office. Report to the Ranking Member, Committee on Homeland Security and Governmental Affairs, United States Senate: Rural hospital closures (p. 1). Published December, 2020. https://www.gao.gov/assets/gao-21-93.pdf

88. Sharma H, Baten R, Ullrich F, et al. Trends in nursing home closures in nonmetropolitan and metropolitan counties in the United States, 2008-2018. RUPRI Center for Rural Health Policy Analysis. Published February, 2021. https://rupri.public-health.uiowa.edu/publications/policybriefs/2021/Rural%20NH%20Closure.pdf

89. Health Resources and Services Administration. Rural community programs. Accessed June, 2022. https://www.hrsa.gov/rural-health/community/index.html

90. Rural Health Information Hub. Rural tribal health. Accessed May 31, 2022. https://www .ruralhealthinfo.org/topics/rural-tribal-health

91. The American Nurses Association's white paper on nurse staffing: clinical and economic benefits of appropriate staffing. *MCN Am J Matern Child Nurs.* 2016;41(3):139. doi:10.1097/NMC.0000000000000242

92. Kasprak J. California RN staffing ratio law. *OLR Research Report.* Published February 10, 2004. https://www.cga.ct.gov/2004/rpt/2004-r-0212.htm

93. Serratt T. California's nurse-to-patient ratios, part 3: eight years later, what do we know about patient level outcomes? *J Nurs Adm*. 2013;43(11):581-585. doi:10.1097/01.NNA.0000434505.69428.eb

94. Everhart D, Neff D, Al-Amin M, Nogle J, Weech-Maldonado R. The effects of nurse staffing on hospital financial performance: competitive versus less competitive markets. *Health Care Manage Rev*. 2013;38(2):146-155. doi:10.1097/HMR.0b013e318257292b

95. Welton JM. Hospital nursing workforce costs, wages, occupational mix, and resource utilization. *J Nurs Adm*. 2011;41(7-8):309-314. doi:10.1097/NNA.0b013e3182250a2b

96. Dean G. Half of nurses said they're thinking of quitting the profession within 2 years in a survey. Higher pay and better staffing could convince them to stay. *Business Insider*. Published October 19, 2021. https://www.businessinsider.com/nurse-shortage-labor-quit-healthcare-hospital-jobs-employment-shiftmed-survey-2021-10

97. Farmer B. More nurses are quitting their jobs to try a lucrative stint as a traveling nurse. *National Public Radio*. Published October 18, 2021. https://www.npr.org/2021/10/18/1046952444/more-nurses-are-quitting-to-try-a-lucrative-stint-as-a-traveling-nurse

98. Brantley E, Bodas M, Chen C, et al. House-passed build back better would bolster public health infrastructure, health workforce. *Health Affairs*. Accessed November 22, 2021. doi:10.1377/hblog20211121.674613. https://www.healthaffairs.org/do/10.1377/forefront.20211121.674613/full/

99. Pham HH, Greiner A. The importance of primary care—and of measuring it. *Health Affairs*. Published August 6, 2019. doi:10.1377/hblog20190802.111704

100. Agency for Healthcare Research and Quality. Primary care workforce facts and stats. Accessed July, 2018. https://www.ahrq.gov/research/findings/factsheets/primary/pcworkforce/index.html

101. OECD statistics. Physicians by categories. https://stats.oecd.org/Index.aspx?DataSetCode=HEALTH_STAT#

102. Rotenstein LS, Holmgren AJ, Downing NL, Bates DW. Differences in total and after-hours electronic health record time across ambulatory specialties. *JAMA Intern Med*. 2021;181(6):863-865.

103. Nath B, Williams B, Jeffery MM, et al. Trends in electronic health record inbox messaging during the COVID-19 pandemic in an ambulatory practice network in New England. *JAMA Netw Open*. 2021;4(10):e2131490. doi:10.1001/jamanetworkopen.2021.31490

104. Berg S. Physician burnout: which medical specialties feel the most stress. *American Medical Association*. Published January 21, 2020. https://www.ama-assn.org/practice-management/physician-health/physician-burnout-which-medical-specialties-feel-most-stress

105. Institute of Medicine (US) Committee on the Future of Primary Care; Donaldson MS, Yordy KD, et al., eds. The value of primary care. In *Primary Care: America's Health in a New Era*. National Academies Press; 1996. https://www.ncbi.nlm.nih.gov/books/NBK232636/

106. Medical Group Management Association. New MGMA research finds physician compensation increased in 2019. Published May 20, 2020. https://www.mgma.com/news-insights/press/new-mgma-research-finds-physician-compensation-inc

107. National Committee for Quality Assurance. Patient-centered medical home (PCMH). https://www.ncqa.org/programs/health-care-providers-practices/patient-centered-medical-home-pcmh/

108. Grumbach K, Bodenheimer T, Cohen D, Phillips RL, Stange KC, Westfall JM. Revitalizing the U.S. primary care infrastructure. *N Engl J Med*. 2021;385(13):1156-1158. doi:10.1056/NEJMp2109700

Insurance

The Basics and Background of Insurance

What Is Insurance and Why Have It?

The logic behind insurance is twofold. First, money should be set aside in small increments over time to spread out the potential cost of an unexpected large expense. Second, your money should be pooled with others' money to further spread out large costs across a population, so that, ideally, no person has to face large costs they cannot afford. For example, most states require minimum liability auto insurance. The benefit to insured individuals is that, as long as you make monthly payments, your accidents are (partially) covered. The benefit to the insurance company is that it gets to keep your monthly payments if those accidents never happen. The benefit to society is that no one is left completely uncovered, and the finances of a few car crashes seem more trivial when the costs are spread out among thousands of people.

Metaphors are useful, but limited. A car is not equivalent to a human, and society's values make us wary of simply making people deal with the severe consequences of illness and death because of the lack of ability to afford care. Our health is a much bigger deal than any car could ever be.

How Do You Get Insurance?

In order to understand what insurance coverage is available or optimal, there are several questions to ask:

■ Are you in a government-covered (ie, entitled) group?
■ Are you employed, and does your employer or union offer health insurance plans?
■ Do you have a spouse/parent who can add you to their coverage?
■ What state and county do you live in?
■ Do you have ongoing, expected health care spending?
■ How much money do you make?

There are many paths to getting insurance, most of which are not available to everyone. In this chapter, we will walk through the types of insurance out there (both public and private). First, let's review some basic insurance terms and concepts.

Insurance Terms and Concepts

An individual enrolled in a health insurance plan is known as a beneficiary or member. The insurance company charges the beneficiary a monthly fee, called a premium. When the beneficiary receives health care services, the insurance company will then reimburse that clinician, clinic, or hospital on behalf of the beneficiary—this is why an insurance company can also be called a "payer." In addition, the individual has to share costs for some of her care with her insurer, thus paying "out of pocket."

Cost-sharing comes in different flavors (Figure 2.1):

■ **Deductible:** A fixed dollar lower threshold. Until the beneficiary's health care costs have hit this threshold, she has to pay all costs out of pocket. For example, if the deductible is $500, the first $500 spent on health care in that year will be paid by the beneficiary. For anything over $500, the insurance may cover the costs completely or require other cost-sharing.

Understanding Cost-Sharing

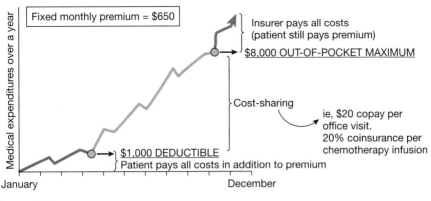

Figure 2.1

- **Copayment (or "copay"):** Fixed dollar amount the beneficiary must pay for certain services. For instance, a beneficiary might have to pay $20 for each appointment, or $10 for each medication refill.
- **Coinsurance:** A percentage of the bill rather than a fixed amount. For instance, a beneficiary might pay 20% of a hospital bill.
- **Out-of-Pocket Maximum:** The fixed dollar upper threshold. Once the beneficiary's health costs have hit this threshold, she doesn't have to pay anything else. No matter what other health care services she receives that year, the insurance company will pay 100% of the cost. For example, the out-of-pocket max in 2021 for a Marketplace plan is $8,550 for an individual and $17,100 for a family.[1]

In addition to cost, a patient might be thinking about *who* they can see. Most private insurance plans contract with a particular subset of physicians and care facilities, called a provider network. Care received from the list is in-network—and generally covered—whereas care from providers not on that list is out-of-network and only partially covered with higher cost-sharing—or not covered at all. Some provider networks are broad, allowing beneficiaries a lot of choice in whom they see, but many are "narrow," meaning they restrict who the insurance company will reimburse for services (so the patient is on the hook for the total cost). Insurance companies use this restriction as a way to keep spending down, only contracting when they get favorable rates from the physicians and hospitals. However, these narrow networks may contain unexpected and enormous omissions; for instance, in 2015, a study[2] found that 30% of plans on the Federal Marketplace did not cover *any* emergency physicians—a problem that could leave patients with a lot of out-of-network, or "surprise," bills (see Section "Surprise Billing" in Chapter 6).

Cost-Sharing

Cost-sharing shifts some patient costs away from monthly premiums, which are prospective and distributed, to payment at the point-of-service, like an office visit or a magnetic resonance imaging (MRI). With cost-sharing, not only do patients who use more resources take on more of the cost burden, but that cost burden is both visible to them and somewhat under their control (ie, they can choose not to use the service).

Cost-sharing is an important mechanism for influencing behavior by insurance companies as well as policy-makers (see Section "Rationing" in Chapter 3). The goal is to put patients' "skin in the game" so they will act like savvy consumers to use less and less expensive care, same as someone who might buy a cheaper cell phone when they are footing the bill than if their workplace is. This is at least partially the concept behind high-deductible plans and is a popular conservative health policy strategy (see Section "Reform" in Chapter 6).

But does it work as intended? The research suggests not. In the 1970s, the RAND Health Insurance Experiment randomized approximately 2,700 families into insurance plans with variable amounts of cost-sharing.[3] RAND found that although those with high cost-sharing *did* reduce their use of services, they did so by simply getting less care, regardless of the preventive nature, quality, or effectiveness of that care, nor did they shop around when they did seek treatment. Although RAND found health outcomes to be roughly the same regardless of cost-sharing, recent research suggests that cost-sharing, by influencing patients to cut back on high-value as well as low-value medications, may lead to higher mortality.[4]

Progressive policy-makers aim to reduce cost-sharing; for instance, the Medicare4All proposal would eliminate cost-sharing (unlike the current, traditional Medicare). This is similar to the United Kingdom, where out-of-pocket spending is very limited. However, it is important to note that the United Kingdom does use other strategies to limit the use of cost-ineffective or low-value care: notably, with the National Institute of Care Excellence, which decides whether to cover treatments at all, based on cost-effectiveness. Such limitations on patient choice would likely cause an uproar in the culture of the United States.

If you want to use cost-sharing, the question is how to do so in a way that doesn't disincentivize the kind of care you want patients to get (a practical concern) nor overburdens people with serious illness (a moral concern). If you want to eliminate cost-sharing, the question is what other mechanism you'll use to ration low-value care. Either way, you'll need to identify what care is high versus low value, and in what circumstances—which is not always clear-cut.

Utilization Management

Historically, providers of medical services (clinicians and hospitals, typically) have been paid a fee for each service they provided. In the 1970s and 1980s, both available services as well as the fees rose, resulting in rising health care costs. In response, insurance companies (and government paid insurance) no longer just paid whatever bill was sent to them: they began to use tactics to ensure those bills were smaller and the services were "justified." These tactics are called utilization management, or managed care.

Some examples of utilization management include:

1. Only covering services from certain providers
2. Prior authorization or pre-authorization, meaning the insurance company must approve a service (such as an MRI, or an expensive medication) before the patient can get it. Typically, this means paperwork for the clinician, a wait for the patient, and strict rules from the insurance company about who qualifies for the service.
3. Higher cost-sharing for more expensive services
4. Requiring a referral from a primary care clinician before seeing a specialist
5. Putting caps on payment for hospital care (see Section "Understanding Reimbursement" in Chapter 3)

Managed care is everywhere, even if it doesn't always go by that name. Health maintenance organizations (HMOs) are common forms of private insurance, which tend to more strictly use the above tactics; one prominent example is Kaiser Permanente (see HMOs and Kaiser later in this chapter). The government contracts out much of Medicaid and Medicare to private managed care insurers, all of which use utilization management tactics (see Section "Medicare" in this chapter and Section "Medicare Advantage" in Chapter 3).

Utilization management lowers costs, but it also creates a headache for both clinicians (who have to submit more paperwork to justify their services) and patients (who have to jump through hoops and wait for approvals).

Trade-offs

There is a trade-off between premiums and benefits; generally, the more you pay monthly, the better benefits and/or the more choice you get. For instance, plans with broad provider networks and less cost-sharing tend to have higher premiums.[5] On the flip side, a high-deductible plan with a narrow network should have a much lower premium. In general, someone with ongoing, predictable health needs—say, someone with chronic conditions—would be better off choosing the higher premium plan. Yet, without price transparency or the ability to predict your own health care needs, it's impossible for patients to know whether they're getting the trade-off that they prefer—so they may just choose the cheapest. Plus, the fine print of insurance coverage is so complicated that even a careful consumer might not truly understand all of the trade-offs. As the *New York Times* puts it, "People carefully weighing two plans—choosing a higher monthly cost or a larger deductible—have no idea that they may also be picking a much worse price when they later need care."[6]

Insurance Churn

Because of moves, job changes, or income loss, most people don't stick with the same health insurance for long. Nearly 25% of low-income adults leave their plans each year (including losing coverage or switching to Medicaid)[7]—and similar turnover affects Medicare Advantage (MA) plans, which sees a range of 8% to 33% changeup in their patients each year.[8,9] This churn is not only a burden and stress on patients; it also disincentivizes up-front investments by insurance plans in preventive health, chronic disease management, and new medical technologies, which often take years or decades to reap cost-savings (not to mention health outcomes)—meaning some other insurer is likely to reap the benefit of the investment. This problem has implications for delivery innovations and alternative payment models (APMs) as well.

What Did the Affordable Care Act Change About Insurance Coverage (Mostly)?

The Affordable Care Act (ACA) passed in 2010, and most of its provisions went into effect in 2014. Much of what has been popular about the law has been consumer protections with insurance. The law is 2,000 pages long, but let's highlight a few major changes in insurance regulations. (For a more comprehensive review of the legacy of the ACA, see Section "Legacy of the ACA at 10 Years" in Chapter 6.)

- **Preexisting Conditions:** Barred insurers from denying coverage because of preexisting health conditions. This has been a very popular regulation.
- **Community Rating:** Barred insurers from charging higher premiums based on current or projected health status. Insurers can only consider age, geographic location, family composition, and tobacco use when setting premiums.[a]

---

[a]This regulation brought all insurance in line with employer-sponsored insurance, which has always been community rated.

- **Lifetime Limits:** Barred lifetime limits. It used to be that an insurer might stop paying *anything* after a certain limit was reached (say, $2 million)—and there were news stories about medically complex, ill babies hitting their lifetime limit by 4 months of age. Since 2014, there is no such limit.
- **Dependent Coverage:** Adult offspring can stay on their parents' insurance as dependents until age 26.
- **Medical Loss Ratio (MLR):** The MLR is the percentage of your insurance premium that pays for health care as opposed to administrative costs, marketing, salaries, overhead, and company profits. Previously, the MLR was unregulated, and the percentage paid out on health costs could be rather low. The ACA requires insurers to keep MLR at 85+% for large group insurers and 80+% for small group insurers.
- **Essential Benefits:**[b] Requires a minimum of broad benefits to be covered by all plans. This list is actually pretty complicated, can vary over time, and states can add their own requirements, too. The idea is that insurers cannot sell plans that won't pay for "essential" aspects of care, like pregnancy or prescription drugs, and that generally insurance you buy on the individual market should be about as robust as what someone would get through their employer.
- Care labeled as "preventive services" cannot have cost-sharing applied to it.[c] For example, the list includes screening mammograms and immunizations.

The ACA effectively required these regulations not by banning all noncompliant plans but rather by restricting such noncompliant plans to be sold for only a 3-month duration. However, in 2018, the Trump administration changed this regulation to allow noncompliant plans to be sold for a year and then renewed for 3 years. So you can still find plans out there that do not meet these requirements (see Section "Short-Term Limited Duration Insurance Plans" later in this chapter).

Insurance: Types and Options

Public Insurance

Thirty-four percent of Americans receive health insurance through one of the following government programs: Medicare, Medicaid, Children's Health Insurance Program (CHIP), TRICARE (for active duty military members), and the Veterans Health Administration (VHA; for veterans) (Figure 2.2).[10]

---

[b]However, older plans not meeting these requirements could be grandfathered in if beneficiaries liked them and wanted to keep them.
[c]These services must have an "A" or "B" recommendation from the U.S. Preventive Services Task Force.

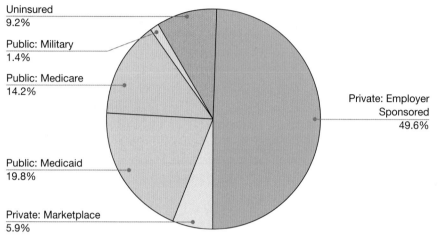

Figure 2.2

Let's go through these programs

Medicare

Medicare is a federal program established in 1965 to insure the elderly and some disabled individuals. It is the largest insurer in the nation—meaning the policies and payment regulations set by Medicare have an enormous impact on how health care is run in general.

Who is covered?

To be eligible for coverage, a person must:

Be at least 65 years old—plus have been a U.S. citizen or permanent resident for more than 5 years, and have (or have a spouse who has) paid Medicare taxes for at least 10 years

If you are under 65, you can only be on Medicare if you also:

- Are permanently disabled and have been receiving Social Security disability benefits for at least the previous 2 years
- Have amyotrophic lateral sclerosis (ALS) and receive Social Security disability benefits
- Need continuous hemodialysis or a kidney transplant
- Developed health conditions following environmental hazard exposure in an emergency declaration area after June 17, 2009.

About 15% of Medicare beneficiaries are under age 65.[11]

What coverage do they get (and not get)?

Medicare coverage has four parts:

Part A: Inpatient insurance, covering stays in hospitals and nursing homes, posthospital home health care, and hospice. These benefits, however, have a limit on the number of days they will pay for in a facility, and they are subject to cost-sharing. Everyone who has Medicare has Part A.

Part B: Outpatient insurance, including coverage for clinician services, preventive services, and home health care. These benefits are also subject to cost-sharing. Most people have Part B, but it is not required.

Part C (More Commonly Called Medicare Advantage): A private insurance alternative to Parts A and B. Established in 1997, MA allows beneficiaries to enroll in a private insurance plan, which must cover all regular Medicare benefits—and may cover more (such as dental or better hearing aid coverage) or offer reduced cost-sharing, but might also have more limits on which clinicians you can see. Medicare pays these private insurers a fixed amount per month, per beneficiary. About 26 million—or 42% of Medicare beneficiaries—were in an MA plan in 2021, with over 3,000 plans on offer nationwide.[12]

Part D: Added in 2005, this is a prescription drug benefit. Part D is voluntary and operates through contracted private insurers, with premiums based on income. The program is subsidized, particularly for low-income beneficiaries.

Parts A and B are often called "traditional Medicare," in contrast to MA.

How much do individuals pay?

Medicare is not free. Some of the costs are standard, and some vary based on income as well as which Part D plan you choose and how many medications you take. In 2016, the average out-of-pocket spending per beneficiary was $5,460.[13] In traditional, Part A and Part B Medicare, there is no out-of-pocket maximum. However, MA plans do have an out-of-pocket maximum, which was $7,550[d] in 2021 (see the Note on the Inflation Reduction Act at the beginning of this book).[14] Let's look at an example of how those costs add up, for an example patient *Linda* who was hospitalized and started cancer treatment (Table 2.1).

Most beneficiaries access additional—or supplemental—insurance to reduce their out-of-pocket expenses. Options include:

- Employer-sponsored retirement benefits
- Medigap: voluntary insurance offered by private insurers to cover cost-sharing (You can't have this with MA.)

---

[d]But only for in-network services! For all out-of-network plus in-network, the max is $11,300.

Table 2.1 Example of Medicare Costs

Occurrence	Medicare coverage	Linda's cost with Medicare
Part A (with one hospitalization in a year)	Everything above the $1,484 deductible	$1,484 deductible No premium cost[a]
Post-acute care stay after hospital (25 d)	Full coverage for days 1-20; $185/d cost-sharing for days 21-100	$185 × 4 d = $740
Part B monthly premium	–	$170[b] × 12 mo = $1,782
Part B deductible	–	$203
Doctor's office visits	All but 20% coinsurance	$20[c] × 8 visits = $160
Lab tests	All but 20% coinsurance	$20[c] × 3 blood draws = $60
Chemo infusion	All but 20% coinsurance	$1,200[c]
Physical therapy visits	All but 20% coinsurance	$20[c] × 6 visits = $120
Part D monthly premium	Big variability here	$33[c] × 12 mo = $396 (but the actual range is $5-207 per month)
Part D deductible	Big variability here	$480[c]
Medications	*Big* variability here, but often ~$10/mo for generics and $40-$100 for brand names	$2,000 for all medications[d]
Patient's annual out-of-pocket health care costs		$8,625

[a]Linda pays no premium for Part A because she paid Medicare taxes as part of her employment for over 10 years. If she hadn't, then she would have to pay a monthly premium, which is $471 in 2021.
[b]Most people pay this standard premium, although there is an additional cost for higher income beneficiaries. In 2022, the premium rose by the most it ever has in a single year, in large part because of a single medication (see Chapter 6).
[c]Estimated costs for simplicity. For Part D we used the averages.
[d]This is hard to estimate and has a huge range. ~1.2 million Medicare beneficiaries have out-of-pocket drug costs over $2,000. Given cancer therapy, we figure Linda would be in this group, and we chose $2,000 for simplicity.
Sources: Adapted from Medicare.gov. Costs. https://www.medicare.gov/your-medicare-costs/medicare-costs-at-a-glance; Kaiser Family Foundation. An overview of the Medicare Part D prescription drug benefit. Published October 2021. https://www.kff.org/medicare/fact-sheet/an-overview-of-the-medicare-part-d-prescription-drug-benefit/; Cubanski J. Key facts about Medicare Part D enrollment, premiums, and cost sharing in 2021. https://www.kff.org/medicare/issue-brief/key-facts-about-medicare-part-d-enrollment-premiums-and-cost-sharing-in-2021/; Cubanski J, Rae M, Young K, Damico Anthony. How does prescription drug spending and use compare across large employer plans, Medicare Part D, and Medicaid? *Kaiser Family Foundation.* Published May 20, 2019. https://www.kff.org/medicare/issue-brief/how-does-prescription-drug-spending-and-use-compare-across-large-employer-plans-medicare-part-d-and-medicaid/

- Medicaid
- VA coverage

How do clinicians get paid?

See Chapter 3 for more explanation. In brief, Medicare sets a standard fee schedule for each service (ie, FFS). On the other hand, CMS pays MA (Part C) plans, a fee per beneficiary (adjusted for how sick those beneficiaries are), and then the plan can negotiate payment rates with different health care providers.

How is the program financed?

Two trust funds managed by the U.S. Treasury hold money earmarked for Medicare. The Hospital Insurance Trust Fund is funded largely by payroll taxes and mostly pays out Part A benefits. The Supplemental Medicare Trust Fund is funded largely by premiums as well as funds authorized by Congress, and mostly pays out for Part B and Part D.[15] Interestingly, beneficiaries only contribute 15% of the funding through their premiums.[16] Since 1965, spending has far exceeded what beneficiaries have contributed in taxes.[17]

Medicaid and CHIP

Medicaid is a joint federal–state program established in 1965 to insure the poor. CHIP (sometimes referred to as S-CHIP, for State Children's Insurance Program) is a joint federal–state program established in 1997 to insure low-income children. Unlike with Medicare, which is a federal program with one set of standards across the nation, Medicaid and CHIP eligibility and reimbursement policies vary quite a bit by state (Table 2.2).

Table 2.2 Medicaid and CHIP Enrollment

	Pre-ACA Medicaid and CHIP average enrollment	Medicaid and CHIP average enrollment in May 2021	% change
United States	56.5 million	82.8 million	+44%
Texas	4.2 million	5.0 million	+19%
California	7.6 million	12.8 million	+65%

CHIP, Children's Health Insurance Program.
Source: Adapted from Kaiser Family Foundation. Total monthly Medicaid/CHIP enrollment and pre-ACA enrollment. Published February 2022. https://www.kff.org/health-reform/state-indicator/total-monthly-medicaid-and-chip-enrollment/?currentTimeframe=0&sortModel=%7B%22colId%22:%22Location%22,%22sort%22:%22asc%22%7D

Who is covered?

To be eligible for Medicaid, a person must belong to one of the following "categorically eligible" groups:

1. Children
2. Parents with dependent children
3. Pregnant women
4. People with severe disabilities
5. Seniors (meaning that many Medicaid recipients are "dual eligibles," that is, they receive both Medicare and Medicaid)

Note that "low-income non-disabled adults" are not on the list. Note, too, that Medicaid is extremely important for people who do have long-term disabilities, whose care needs (including in-home and nursing home care) and costs are often so high that Medicaid is an absolutely necessary lifeline. People with disabilities make up 15% of the Medicaid population but account for 42% of spending.[18]

In addition to being in one of the categorically eligible groups, Medicaid beneficiaries must have low income. States must cover citizens in these groups who have incomes below thresholds based on the federal poverty level (FPL; in 2022, $13,590 annually for an individual or $27,750 for a family of four[19]), and there are no enrollment limits—if a state happens to have an unusually high number of residents who fit in these groups, the state must cover them all. States have the authority to be *more* generous: they can cover any low-income individual even if not in one of the above groups, and they can allow eligibility at higher incomes, as Massachusetts does.

Starting in 2014, the ACA mandated a large expansion of Medicaid to include anyone with an income of 138% or less of the FPL. However, this only applies to states that chose to expand (and accept more federal money for) Medicaid (Figure 2.3).

How much did expansion increase coverage? Let's look at an example, between California and Texas. California and Texas have very different income cutoffs for being on Medicaid, and Texas did not expand Medicaid, whereas California did. Like all states, the income cutoffs are based on a percentage of the FPL. In California, the maximum allowable income for a single parent of three children is 138% of FPL, or $38,295 annually.[20] In Texas, that cutoff is 14% of FPL, or $3,885 annually[21] (Note that there are asset limits, too, not just income!) (Table 2.2).

Status of Medicaid Expansion as of November 2021

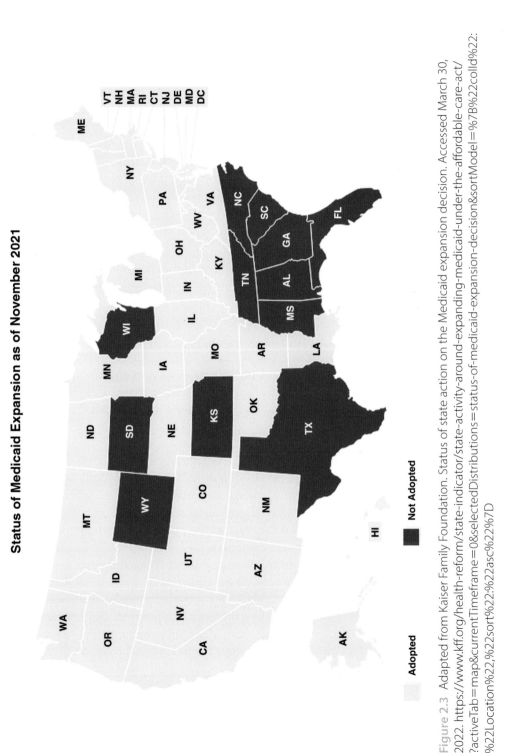

Figure 2.3 Adapted from Kaiser Family Foundation. Status of state action on the Medicaid expansion decision. Accessed March 30, 2022. https://www.kff.org/health-reform/state-indicator/state-activity-around-expanding-medicaid-under-the-affordable-care-act/?activeTab=map&currentTimeframe=0&selectedDistributions=status-of-medicaid-expansion-decision&sortModel=%7B%22colId%22:%22Location%22,%22sort%22:%22asc%22%7D

Coverage options for kids

CHIP's purpose is to expand insurance to children who aren't eligible for Medicaid coverage. However, there are no hard-and-fast rules for eligibility; states have broad authority to set their own rules. As of 2018, Medicaid covered about 37 million children in the nation and CHIP covered 9 million.[22]

What coverage do they get (and not get)?

Medicaid programs are required to offer minimum benefits, though some states choose to offer more. Rather than go through a list of required coverage, let's mention the services that Medicaid provides outsized coverage for across the population:

- Medicaid pays for 43% of all births.[23]
- Medicaid pays for 51% of all long-term nursing home and home health care.[24]
- Medicaid pays for 25% of all behavioral health spending, including substance use treatment.[25]

How much do individuals pay?

Thirty-five states include some cost-sharing for adults. Although the details and amount vary from state to state, the total amount remains low. In 2020, for someone at or below the FPL, the most they could be charged was $4 for a drug prescription, $75 for a hospital stay, and $4 for a doctor's visit.[26]

How does the program pay providers?

Similar to Medicare, Medicaid pays providers a standard fee based on service provided; these vary by state but average to only 72% of what Medicare will pay.[27] As of 2016, about 81% of Medicaid patients were in a managed care plan[28]; similar to MA, these managed care plans are paid an annual fee per beneficiary by the state, and then they can set their own rates with providers.

Many complain about low reimbursement by Medicaid, and in fact fewer physicians will accept new Medicaid patients—about 70%, compared to 90% for private insurance[29]—though reasons for this may be more complicated than just payment.

Medicaid payment to hospitals is a bit more complicated, and hospitals who admit a higher than average percent of Medicaid patients are paid a supplemental fee called a disproportionate share hospital (DSH) payment.[30]

How is the program financed?

Medicaid is a federal–state (and sometimes county) partnership. The Federal Medical Assistance Percentage (FMAP) is the amount contributed by the federal government to the states (see Section "Setting Payments to States in Medicaid: Federal Medical Assistance Program (FMAP)" in Chapter 6). The

FMAP ranges from a low of 56% to a high of 84% in 2021.[31] For some states, Medicaid is both their largest expenditure as well as—because of the FMAP— their top revenue source.[32]

Veterans Health Administration

VHA is a component of the U.S. Department of Veterans Affairs that provides medical care to veterans and their families at low or no cost. As of 2020, the VHA enrolled 9.2 million beneficiaries, which is slightly less than half of all veterans.[33] Veterans become eligible for these health benefits based on disability (stemming from their service), service history, and income level. Many veterans also have other insurance beyond the VHA, such as through employers, Medicare, or Medicaid.

Benefits include outpatient and hospital care as well as medications—all through VHA sites—as well as medical equipment and long-term care such as supported housing. Most veterans pay nothing for their care,[e] but those without disability or low-income status pay copays such as $15 for primary care visits, $50 for MRIs, and $300 to $1,500 for up to 3 months of hospital care.[34]

All providers are employed by the federal government as salaried employees—similar to the National Health Service in the United Kingdom, and in contrast to the way providers are typically reimbursed through other insurance systems. (Without getting too into the weeds, the VHA also covers some services obtained at non-VHA facilities.) The VHA is financed entirely through federal funding and cost $69 billion in 2017.[35] (Using simple math, that's about $7,532 per VA beneficiary; compare to the average US expenditure of $12,530 per person).[36]

TRICARE

TRICARE is a Department of Defense program that provides care to active duty military members, some retirees, and their dependents, covering about 9.6 million worldwide.[37] Similar to the VHA, TRICARE covers comprehensive outpatient, hospital, and medication care, but all through the TRICARE system. Active duty members and their families pay nothing for care. Retirees are subject to copays such as $150 to $366 annual enrollment fees for an individual, $31 for a primary care visit, and $158 for a hospital admission.[38] Also like the VHA, all providers are employed by the federal government, and the program is financed through federal funding. (And, also like the VHA, TRICARE will pay for some private medical services.)

---

[e]Enrollees with greater than 10% disability rating have no copay, and the majority of VHA enrollees have this rating.

Private Insurance

Looking back at our insurance chart from the beginning of this section, we see that private insurance covers about 55% of all Americans and represents about 31% of spending. People can purchase private insurance independently (typically through a Marketplace), but most receive it through their employers. Private insurance is regulated primarily at the state level, rather than at the national level like Medicare.

(Private) Insurance Types—Organization Formats

In the not-so-distant past, patients directly paid their doctors for services rendered. Not so today. The development and change of health insurance over time (since the first hospital insurance was offered in 1929) is an interesting story, but here we will just focus on the current offerings of insurance plans. At their most basic, all organization formats can be thought of as a different way of handling the trade-offs between up-front costs, coverage, and restrictions on patient choice of provider.

Keep in mind that some public insurance—through MA and managed Medicaid plans—are administered through private companies and thus include the following formats.

A very basic comparison of some major private insurance plan types:

- **Health Maintenance Organization:** HMOs tend to keep premiums low by raising deductibles and narrowly restricting which providers they cover in-network and requiring a referral from a primary care physician (PCP) to see a specialist. HMOs gained a lot of traction in the 1990s, but also angered a lot of patients and providers by overly limiting care.
- **Preferred Provider Organization (PPO):** These tend to have higher premiums but with lower deductibles and copays, and more flexibility in terms of which physicians you can see.
- **High-Deductible Health Plans:** These are plans with an annual deductible of at least $1,400 for an individual or $2,800 for a family. Typically, the monthly premium is lower. These plans are often combined with pre–tax saving accounts that can only be used for health-related expenses, called flexible spending accounts (FSAs) or health spending accounts (HSAs). These plans put a lot of cost-sharing up-front for beneficiaries and are a common strategy for putting patients' "skin in the game."

The specifics of what each type of plan covers are even more variable, though. An insurance company such as Cigna may have hundreds of different options for PPO plans, for instance.

Employer-Sponsored Insurance

The United States is unlike other countries in that so many people get their insurance through their workplace. This strange relationship between health care and employers arose during World War II, after the federal government enacted a freeze on wage increases in the private industry. In response, employers improved their nonwage benefits, including health insurance, for employees and their families. This arrangement of employer-sponsored insurance (ESI) spread even more rapidly when the Internal Revenue Service (IRS) ruled that employer payments for insurance weren't taxable (ie, a tax break for ESI beneficiaries).[39] ESI became the predominant method of obtaining insurance in the United States, representing 70% of insured Americans in 2009—although this fell to 50% by 2019,[40] because the ACA expanded the pool of the insured, making it easier to get insurance through the Marketplaces or Medicaid.

The majority of employers buy insurance from a private insurance company, though, increasingly, large employers will "self-insure," meaning the employer acts as the insurer by itself taking the premiums and assuming financial risk for pay-outs, though it often still pays a third-party administrator to handle premiums and claims.[10] Other employers usually work with a broker to price different insurance options—like HMOs and PPOs from different insurers—and the employee can select from one of these employer-approved plans.

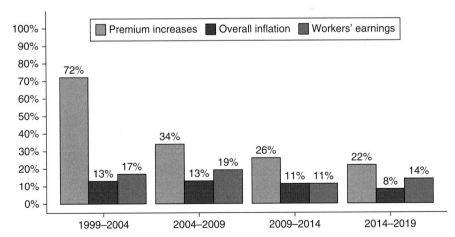

Cumulative Premium Increases, Inflation, and Earnings for Covered Workers With Family Coverage, 1999-2019

Figure 2.4 Adapted from KFF Employer Health Benefits Survey, 2018-2019, Kaiser/HRET survey of employer sponsored health benefits, 1999-2017; Bureau of Labor Statistics; Consumer Price Index, U.S. City Average of Annual inflation [April-April] 1999-2019; Bureau of Labor Statistics, Seasonally Adjusted. Data from the current employment statistics Survey, 1999-2019 [April-April].

Most plans will also cover a spouse and dependents for an increased payment, though while large employers are required to cover dependent children up to age 26, they are not actually required to cover spouses, nor to pay anything toward these family members' premiums. For employees, premiums are the same across the board (ie, community rated, meaning that the benefit the ACA enacted was one that those with ESI were getting all along).[f] The employer contributes 50% to 90% of the monthly premium, and the employee pays the rest. Employees see reduced wages, as employers must pay less in wages to maintain this benefit; however, neither employees nor employers have to pay income tax on benefits. Thus, though employees have reduced wages, they receive a larger total compensation package.

Unfortunately, with ESI, losing your job means you lose your health insurance, too. Recognizing this risk, the Consolidated Omnibus Budget Reconciliation Act or COBRA was enacted to require employers to allow employees to continue purchasing their ESI for 18 months after job loss. (Though at a much higher cost, because the former employer is no longer subsidizing the premium!)

Pros and cons of ESI

From the employee's standpoint, ESI provides both advantages and disadvantages. The advantages are reduced premiums (because of both the contribution of the employer as well as the economy of scale), and reduced income taxes. The disadvantages are that it reduces your salary—and there's real concern that rising health care costs have been an important cause of wage suppression. Plus, those who lose their job will also lose their health insurance (at the same time that they have less money to pay for any health care costs).

From the insurance company's standpoint, ESI reduces adverse selection (see Chapter 3) and the need for marketing. A group of employees is likely to be both large (meaning a dependable stream of revenue as long as they maintain a relationship with the employer) and relatively healthy[g] (meaning they won't require as much pay-out on their premiums). Although employers do have the clout to reduce premiums from what individual consumers pay, this is still a profitable trade-off for the insurers.

From the employer's standpoint, if you have over 50 employees, the law says you have to provide ESI. Providing good health benefits has long been a way to entice and retain workers—but benefits get increasingly difficult to provide as health costs rise faster than wages. From 2018 to 2019, premiums for a worker's family coverage rose 5%, whereas wages rose 3.4% and inflation rose 2%[41] (Figure 2.4).

---

[f]ESI premiums may (depending on state law) be adjusted by the insurer to account for the claims history of the employer, so an employer with a track record of employees who need lots of medical care may have to pay a higher premium. Thus, insurance for employees of mining companies is usually more expensive than those of a health food store.
[g]Compared to a similar-sized group of unemployed individuals.

From society's standpoint, ESI is beneficial in that it can insure a large number of citizens without the government directly involved, which is why expanding ESI was originally a conservative policy idea. It's problematic, though, because of the ESI tax subsidy (workers pay taxes only on their wages, not their benefits). Because ESI is paid with pretax dollars, it means that (a) society misses out on those taxes (about $273 billion each year![42]), and (b) those with ESI get more bang for their buck, in contrast to those who purchase insurance outside of employment.

ACA Marketplaces

Millions of Americans can't obtain insurance through their employers or the government—think of the self-employed, early retirees, the nonpoor unemployed, and those working for companies that don't offer ESI—and must turn to the individual market for coverage. Americans could always purchase private insurance, but it was confusing to find and compare plans, and might even be totally unavailable if you had preexisting conditions. The ACA established Marketplaces (also known as Exchanges) as portals for purchasing individual (or group, for small businesses) health insurance. Think of a Marketplace like using Travelocity or Priceline to purchase an airplane flight. The Marketplace offers certain private insurance plans under certain conditions, and you can choose the plan that works best for you. Twenty-one states run their own, and the rest are run by the federal government; in 2021, they connected 12 million people to insurance.[43]

Marketplaces offer a variety of plans based on different levels of trade-off between premiums versus cost-sharing. These are in tiers based on metals, that is, "platinum" plans have higher premiums and lower cost-sharing, whereas "bronze" plans have higher cost-sharing but lower premiums. Folks who buy plans through the Marketplaces are also eligible for subsidies if their income levels are between 138% and 400% of the FPL.[h]

In addition, every Marketplace has standardized the following for insurers to make it easier to understand what is being offered and to compare it fairly to other plans:

- Requires plans to use "plain language" and a standardized format to present benefit options
- Requires plans to explain what services have copays and deductibles

---

[h]The lower number of 138% was chosen since anyone under this threshold was supposed to be covered by Medicaid expansion—but, as we know, some states didn't expand Medicaid. Thus, in a terrible irony, someone in Texas who makes 150% of the FPL is eligible for subsidies on the Marketplace, but someone who makes 90% of the FPL is not!

- Assigns a rating to each health plan based on relative quality and price
- Creates a calculator to determine the actual cost of a plan for each person, including tax credits and cost-sharing
- Informs enrollees about their eligibility for Medicaid

The Marketplaces make it significantly easier to find, compare, and purchase insurance with subsidies. However, they don't provide the insurance itself, and the options may not be ideal. The average number of insurers participating in the Marketplaces is 5, ranging from 13 options in Wisconsin to only a single insurer in Delaware.[44,45]

Spotlight on Kaiser Permanente

Kaiser Permanente was founded in 1945 and is now the nation's largest private, nonprofit insurer. People can get Kaiser insurance many ways: through the Marketplace, through their employer, or as a managed plan for public insurance (MA and managed Medicaid). Kaiser isn't just an insurance plan, though—it is integrated coverage *and* delivery, similar to the VA or TRICARE, in which beneficiaries use Kaiser hospitals and clinics, and see clinicians who only work for Kaiser. It is also a managed care plan.

In the next chapter, we talk about alternative payment models and capitation plans (see Section "APMs and Value-Based Payment" in Chapter 3). Kaiser is an extreme form of capitation and of managed care. The Kaiser model aims to eliminate jockeying around reimbursement, to streamline quality and population health improvements, and to reduce low-value care. This has produced mixed results, with success in some areas and failure in others, underscoring how difficult it is to deliver cost-effective and high-quality care.

Short-Term Limited Duration Insurance Plans

The ACA increased consumer protections in the private insurance market, bringing private insurance plans more in line with what you can get through ESI. However, the law didn't outright ban policy elements like failing to cover preexisting conditions or require essential benefits; rather, the ACA banned selling noncompliant plans for longer than 3 months. In 2018, the Trump administration removed this ban, allowing the sale of such "short-term" plans for 12 months, with renewal for up to 36 months. Afterward, enrollment in these plans increased from 2.36 million to 3 million.[46] These plans cannot be sold through a Marketplace, but they can be purchased in most states, and, in one review, all exclude maternity benefits as well as payment based on preexisting conditions.[47] Some call these "junk" plans, and there are congressional efforts to curtail them again.[48]

Does Insurance Even Accomplish What We Want? The Oregon Medicaid Experiment

In this chapter we've reviewed the landscape of health insurance—a benefit that a lot of health policy revolves around getting people access to. But what we really want is for people to be healthy. Should we question whether health insurance advances that aim?

In 2008, Oregon had the funds to increase Medicaid enrollment by 10,000—but the state received 90,000 applications.[4] They decided to assign enrollment by lottery, randomizing who got insurance. That randomization meant that researchers had a pool of data to examine how insurance—specifically *public* insurance—affects both health outcomes and spending. Ideally, insurance should lead to both improved health as well as more utilization of less costly care (ie, primary care) than of more costly care (ie, the ED), because patients are better able to access preventive services and care that manages their conditions before becoming an emergency. But is that really what happens when people get insurance?

In 2013, research on these outcomes was reported, but it was a mixed bag without clear conclusions. In fact, people across the political spectrum have used the results to support opposite conclusions. Findings of the experiment found that Medicaid coverage[49]:

Increased health care use across the board:

- Increased ED usage, at any time of day and for both emergencies and non-emergencies
- Increased office visits by 2.7 visits a year
- Increased hospitalizations by 30%

Decreased the burden of health care bills:

- Eliminated out-of-pocket catastrophic medical bills
- Decreased the likelihood of having unpaid medical bills sent to collections

Some improvements in health status:

- Increased preventive care substantially, including doubling mammograms
- Increased diagnosis of diabetes and depression, including starting medications for these
- Increased self-reported health status
- Did not change objective measures of health (like blood pressure or cholesterol)
- Improved rates of depression by 30%

Percent of the Nonelderly Population That Is Uninsured, by State, 2019

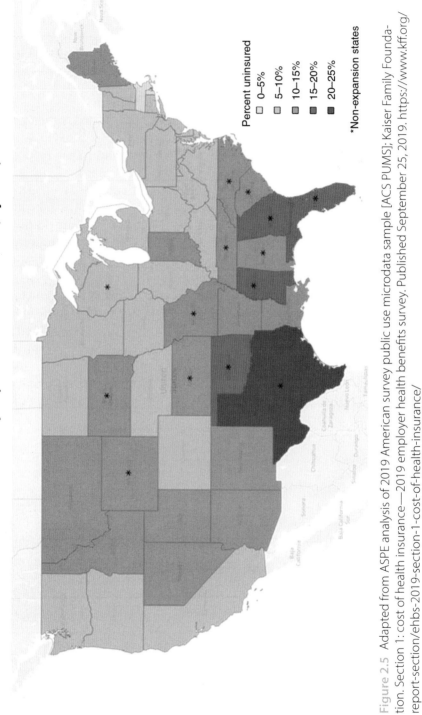

Percent uninsured

- ☐ 0–5%
- ☐ 5–10%
- ☐ 10–15%
- ☐ 15–20%
- ☐ 20–25%

*Non-expansion states

Figure 2.5 Adapted from ASPE analysis of 2019 American survey public use microdata sample [ACS PUMS]; Kaiser Family Foundation. Section 1: cost of health insurance—2019 employer health benefits survey. Published September 25, 2019. https://www.kff.org/report-section/ehbs-2019-section-1-cost-of-health-insurance/

Did not affect employment status

Critics claim these results mean that Medicaid has no positive effect for all its expenditures, and that efforts should focus on getting people on private insurance rather than the "broken system" of public insurance.[50] Supporters, though, say the study had flaws, that some things really did improve, that health outcomes take a long time to achieve after interventions, and that no one submits private insurance to the same scrutiny. And, as two policy experts pointed out, the program was a success in two of the goals of insurance: financial protection and improved access to care.[51]

No Insurance

We would be remiss in discussing the ways people get insurance if we didn't also talk about those who *don't* get insurance. One of the big selling points of the ACA is that it reduced the number of uninsured; the rate of uninsurance fell from 16% in 2010[52] to 9.7% in 2020[53]—though that rate has bumped up slightly since a low in 2016. The gains in insurance were particularly notable for Black, Latino, and Asian Americans, as well as low-income individuals.[54]

In 2020 that still left 31.6 million people—including 5% of children—uninsured.[55] These numbers are higher in states choosing not to expand Medicaid (Figure 2.5). Curiously, in 2019, 57% of uninsured people *did* qualify for Medicaid or subsidized Marketplace insurance coverage.[56]

Through the graphs in Figures 2.6 and 2.7, we can see that the uninsured population, although varied, is mostly made up of low-income, full-time

Characteristics of the Nonelderly Uninsured, 2019

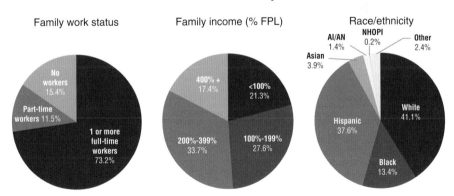

Figure 2.6 AI/AN, American Indian/Alaska Native; FPL, federal poverty level; NHOPI, Native Hawaiians and Other Pacific Islanders. Note: Includes nonelderly individuals ages 0 to 64. Hispanic people may be of any race but are categorized as Hispanic; other groups are all non-Hispanic. The 2019 Census Bureau poverty threshold for a family of three was $20,578. (Adapted from Tolbert J, Orgera K, Damico A. Key facts about the uninsured population. https://www.kff.org/uninsured/issue-brief/key-facts-about-the-uninsured-population/.)

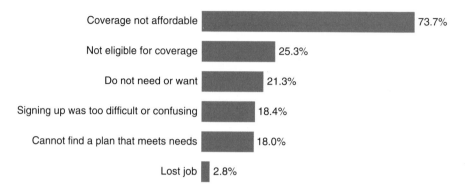

Reasons for Being Uninsured Among Uninsured Nonelderly Adults, 2019

Reason	Percent
Coverage not affordable	73.7%
Not eligible for coverage	25.3%
Do not need or want	21.3%
Signing up was too difficult or confusing	18.4%
Cannot find a plan that meets needs	18.0%
Lost job	2.8%

Figure 2.7 Note: Includes nonelderly individuals ages 18 to 64. Respondents can select multiple options. (Adapted from Tolbert J, Orgera K, Damico A. Key facts about the uninsured population. https://www.kff.org/uninsured/issue-brief/key-facts-about-the-uninsured-population/.)

workers, primarily white and Latino. One quarter of the uninsured are non-citizens.[57] Far and away, the most common reported reason for being uninsured is being unable to afford coverage.

Ten percent of the uninsured say they went without needed medical care because of cost, and 75% report being unable to afford to pay any medical bills.[58] In 2017, uncompensated spending (ie, care never reimbursed because the patients cannot afford to pay them) for the uninsured reached $42.4 billion. Twenty percent of that cost burden fell on the shoulders of the providers who were not compensated, and 80% was ultimately offset through a complex network of government programs, mostly through federal VA and Medicaid funding programs.[59] In this way, society may opt not to "pay now" for universal insurance coverage, but it still "pays later" for the uncompensated care costs that lack of insurance produces.

References

1. HealthCare.Gov. Out of pocket maximum/limit. Accessed March 21, 2022. https://www.healthcare.gov/glossary/out-of-pocket-maximum-limit
2. Dorner SC, Camargo CA Jr, Schuur JD, Raja AS. Access to in-network emergency physicians and emergency departments within federally qualified health plans in 2015. *West J Emerg Med*. 2016;17(1):18-21. doi:10.5811/westjem.2015.12.29188
3. Brook RH, Keeler EB, Lohr KN, et al. The health insurance experiment: a classic RAND study speaks to the current health care reform debate. RAND Corporation; 2006. https://www.rand.org/pubs/research_briefs/RB9174.html

4. Chandra A, Flack E, Obermeyer Z. The health costs of cost-sharing. NBER Working Paper Series. Published February 2021. https://www.nber.org/system/files/working_papers/w28439/w28439.pdf

5. Polsky D, Wu B. Provider networks and health plan premium variation. *Health Serv Res.* 2021;56(1):16-24. doi:10.1111/1475-6773.13447

6. Kliff S, Katz J. Hospitals and insurers didn't want you to see these prices. here's why. *The New York Times.* Published August 22, 2021. https://www.nytimes.com/interactive/2021/08/22/upshot/hospital-prices.html

7. Sommers BD, Gourevitch R, Maylone B, Blendon RJ, Epstein AM. Insurance churning rates for low-income adults under health reform: lower than expected but still harmful for many. *Health Aff (Millwood).* 2016;35(10):1816-1824. doi:10.1377/hlthaff.2016.0455

8. Hsieh M, Smith N, Ipakchi N. Are Medicare advantage plans forgetting to close the back door? Provider sponsored plans lead in Medicare advantage member retention. *Health Management Associates.* 2021. https://www.healthmanagement.com/wp-content/uploads/PSP-Churn-2021-In-Focus-5-5-21_HMA.pdf

9. Jacobson G, Neumann T. Medicare advantage plan switching: exception and norm? Kaiser Family Foundation. Published September 20, 2016. Accessed March 30, 2022. https://www.kff.org/report-section/medicare-advantage-plan-switching-exception-or-norm-issue-brief/

10. Nunn R, Parsons J, Shambaugh J. A dozen facts about the economics of the US health-care system. *Brookings.* Published March 10, 2020. https://www.brookings.edu/research/a-dozen-facts-about-the-economics-of-the-u-s-health-care-system/

11. Kaiser Family Foundation. An overview of Medicare. Published February 13, 2019. Accessed March 30, 2022. https://www.kff.org/medicare/issue-brief/an-overview-of-medicare/

12. Freed M, Damico A, Neumann T. Medicare advantage 2022 spotlight: first look. *Kaiser Family Foundation.* Published November 2, 2021. Accessed March 30, 2022. https://www.kff.org/medicare/issue-brief/medicare-advantage-2022-spotlight-first-look/

13. Cubanski J, Koma W, Damico A, Neumann T. How much do Medicare beneficiaries spent out-of-pocket on care? Kaiser Family Foundation. Published November 4, 2019. Accessed March 30, 2022. https://www.kff.org/medicare/issue-brief/how-much-do-medicare-beneficiaries-spend-out-of-pocket-on-health-care/

14. Freed M, Biniek JF, Damico A, Neumann T. Medicare advantage in 2021: premiums, cost-sharing, out of pocket limits, and supplemental benefits. Published June 21, 2021. Accessed March 30, 2022. https://www.kff.org/medicare/issue-brief/medicare-advantage-in-2021-premiums-cost-sharing-out-of-pocket-limits-and-supplemental-benefits/

15. Medicare.gov. How is Medicare funded? Accessed July 4, 2022. https://www.medicare.gov/about-us/how-is-medicare-funded

16. Cubanski J, Neuman T, Freed M. The facts on Medicare spending and financing. *Kaiser Family Foundation.* Published August 20, 2019. https://www.kff.org/medicare/issue-brief/the-facts-on-medicare-spending-and-financing/

17. Steuerle C, Smith K. Social security & Medicare lifetime benefits and taxes: 2021. *Urban Institute.* (pp. 2-3). Published February 15, 2022. https://www.urban.org/research/publication/social-security-medicare-lifetime-benefits-and-taxes-2021

18. Medicaid and CHIP Payment and Access Commission. Medicaid and persons with disabilities. Published March 2012. https://www.macpac.gov/publication/ch-1-medicaid-and-persons-with-disabilities/

19. HealthCare.Gov. Federal poverty level (FPL). 2022. https://www.healthcare.gov/glossary/federal-poverty-level-fpl/

20. California Department of Health Care Services. Do you qualify for Medi-Cal benefits? Published February 28, 2022. https://www.dhcs.ca.gov/services/medi-cal/Pages/DoYouQualifyForMedi-Cal.aspx

21. Medicaid and CHIP Payment and Access Commission. Medicaid and CHIP eligibility. MACStats: Medicaid and CHIP Data Book. (pp. 100-102). Published December 2021. https://www.macpac.gov/wp-content/uploads/2021/12/MACStats-Medicaid-and-CHIP-Data-Book-December-2021.pdf

22. Center on Budget and Policy Priorities. Medicaid works for children. Published January 19, 2018. https://www.cbpp.org/research/health/medicaid-works-for-children

23. Medicaid and CHIP Payment and Access Commission. Medicaid's role in financing maternity care. (p. 5). Published January 2020. https://www.macpac.gov/wp-content/uploads/2020/01/Medicaid%E2%80%99s-Role-in-Financing-Maternity-Care.pdf

24. Reaves EL, Musumeci M. Medicaid and long-term services and supports: a primer. Published December 15, 2015. https://www.kff.org/medicaid/report/medicaid-and-long-term-services-and-supports-a-primer/

25. Medicaid and CHIP Payment and Access Commission. Behavioral health in the Medicaid Program—people, use, and expenditures. Report to Congress on Medicaid and CHIP. (p. 90). Published June 2015. https://www.macpac.gov/publication/behavioral-health-in-the-medicaid-program%E2%80%95people-use-and-expenditures/

26. Brooks T, Roygardner L, Artiga S, et al. Medicaid and CHIP eligibility, enrollment, and cost sharing policies as of January 2020: findings from a 50-state survey. Published March 26, 2020. https://www.kff.org/report-section/medicaid-and-chip-eligibility-enrollment-and-cost-sharing-policies-as-of-january-2020-findings-from-a-50-state-survey-premiums-and-cost-sharing/

27. Masterson L. Medicaid reimbursement, not expansion status, affects Doctors' acceptance of new patients. *HealthCareDive*. Published April 11, 2019. https://www.healthcaredive.com/news/medicaid-reimbursement-not-expansion-status-affects-doctors-acceptance-o/552476/

28. Medicaid and CHIP Payment and Access Commission. Provider payment and delivery systems. https://www.macpac.gov/medicaid-101/provider-payment-and-delivery-systems/

29. Holgash K, Heberlein M. Physician acceptance of new Medicaid patients: what matters and what doesn't. *Health Affairs*. Published April 10, 2019. doi:10.1377/hblog20190401.678690

30. Cunningham P, Rudowitz R, Young K, et al. Understanding Medicaid hospital payments and the impact of recent policy changes. *Kaiser Family Foundation*. Published June 9, 2016. https://www.kff.org/report-section/understanding-medicaid-hospital-payments-and-the-impact-of-recent-policy-changes-issue-brief/

31. Kaiser Family Foundation. Federal Medical Assistance Percentage (FMAP) for Medicaid and multiplier. 2022. https://www.kff.org/medicaid/state-indicator/federal-matching-rate-and-multiplier/?currentTimeframe=0&sortModel=%7B%22colId%22:%22Location%22,%22sort%22:%22asc%22%7D

32. Snyder L, Rudowitz R. Medicaid financing: how does it work and what are the implications? *Kaiser Family Foundation*. Published May 20, 2015. https://www.kff.org/medicaid/issue-brief/medicaid-financing-how-does-it-work-and-what-are-the-implications/

33. Department of Veterans Affairs. Department of Veterans Affairs statistics at a glance. Published June 30, 2021. https://www.va.gov/vetdata/docs/Quickfacts/Stats_at_a_glance_6_30_21.PDF

34. Department of Veterans Affairs. 2022 VA health care copay rates. 2022. https://www.va.gov/health-care/copay-rates/

35. Golding H. Potential spending on veterans' health care, 2018-2028. Congressional Budget Office. Published November 19, 2018. https://www.cbo.gov/system/files/2018-11/54690-presentation_0.pdf

36. Centers for Medicare & Medicaid Services. National Health Expenditure Fact Sheet, 2020. Accessed July 9, 2022. https://www.cms.gov/Research-Statistics-Data-and-Systems/Statistics-Trends-and-Reports/NationalHealthExpendData/NHE-Fact-Sheet

37. Military Health System. TRICARE beneficiary. 2022. https://health.mil/I-Am-A/TRICARE-Beneficiary

38. Military Health System. TRICARE costs and fees 2022. 2022. https://www.tricare.mil/-/media/Files/TRICARE/Publications/Misc/Costs_Sheet_2022.pdf?la=en&hash=3B008AC63D8D50DB7B444B53E 39EC645726B8E84032168EFD5AA0CB06E4F9ECE

39. Blumenthal D. Employer-sponsored health insurance in the United States-origins and implications. *New Engl J Med.* 2006;355(1):82-88.

40. Kaiser Family Foundation. Health insurance coverage of the total population. 2019. https://www.kff.org/other/state-indicator/total-population/?currentTimeframe=0&sortModel=%7B%22colId%22:%22Location%22,%22sort%22:%22asc%22%7D

41. Miller S. More small and midsize firms choose to self-insure. Society for Human Resource Management. Accessed July 29, 2016. https://www.shrm.org/resourcesandtools/hr-topics/benefits/pages/self-insurance-aca.aspx#:~:text=In%202016%2C%2040.7%20percent%20of,Institute%20reported%20in%20February%202018

42. Kaiser Family Foundation. Section 1: cost of health insurance.—2019 employer health benefits survey. Published September 25, 2019. https://www.kff.org/report-section/ehbs-2019-section-1-cost-of-health-insurance/

43. Tax Policy Center. How does the tax exclusion for employer-sponsored health insurance work? Tax Policy Center's Briefing Book. Urban Institute and Brookings Institution. Published 2019. https://www.taxpolicycenter.org/briefing-book/how-does-tax-exclusion-employer-sponsored-health-insurance-work#:~:text=The%20ESI%20exclusion%20will%20cost,the%20single%20largest%20tax%20expenditure.&text=Making%20the%20credit%20refundable%20would,the%20value%20of%20the%20credit

44. Kaiser Family Foundation. Marketplace enrollment, 2014-2022. Published 2022. https://www.kff.org/health-reform/state-indicator/marketplace-enrollment/?currentTimeframe=0&sortModel=%7B%22colId%22:%22Location%22,%22sort%22:%22asc%22%7D

45. Delaware.gov. Highmark increases 2022 Affordable Care Act marketplace premiums. *Delaware News.* Published August 26, 2021. https://news.delaware.gov/2021/08/26/highmark-increases-2022-affordable-care-act-marketplace-premiums/

46. Kaiser Family Foundation. Number of issuers participating in the individual health insurance marketplaces. 2022. https://www.kff.org/other/state-indicator/number-of-issuers-participating-in-the-individual-health-insurance-marketplace

47. Pallone F, Eshoo AG, DeGette D. Shortchanged: how the Trump administration's expansion of junk short-term health insurance plans is putting Americans at risk. US House of Representatives. Published June 2020. https://drive.google.com/file/d/1uiL3Bi9XV0mYnxpyaIMeg_Q-BJaURXX3/view

48. Palanker D, Curran E, Salyards A. Limitations of short-term health plans persist despite predictions that they'd evolve. *To the Point* (blog), Commonwealth Fund. Published July 22, 2020. doi:10.26099/4x6a-bc25

49. Murphy C, Baldwin T. The Supreme Court protected the ACA. Now, let's protect Americans from junk insurance plans. *Health Affairs Blog.* Published July 7, 2021. doi:10.1377/hblog20210707.277695

50. Baicker K, Finkelstein A, Allen H, et al. Oregon health insurance experiment—results. National Bureau of Economic Research. Accessed April 25, 2022. https://www.nber.org/programs-projects/projects-and-centers/oregon-health-insurance-experiment/oregon-health-insurance-experiment-results

51. Roy A. The Medicaid deniers. *National Review.* Published May 14, 2013. https://www.nationalreview.com/2013/05/medicaid-deniers-avik-roy/

52. Kronick R, Bindman A. Protecting finances and improving access to care with Medicaid. *New Engl J Med.* 2013;368(18):1744-1745. doi:10.1056/nejme1302107. https://escholarship.org/uc/item/1vv4s412

53. Cohen RA, Ward BW, Schiller JS. Health insurance coverage: early release of estimates from the National Health Interview Survey, 2010. National Center for Health Statistics. Published June 2011. doi:10.15620/cdc:108816

54. Finegold K, Conmy A, Chu RC, Bosworth A, Sommers, BD. Trends in the U.S. uninsured population, 2010-2020. (Issue Brief No. HP-2021-02). Office of the Assistant Secretary for Planning and Evaluation, U.S. Department of Health and Human Services. Published February 11, 2021. https://aspe.hhs.gov/sites/default/files/private/pdf/265041/trends-in-the-us-uninsured.pdf

55. Cohen RA, Terlizzi EP, Cha AE, Martinez ME. Health insurance coverage: early release of estimates from the National Health Interview Survey, 2020. National Center for Health Statistics. Published August 2021. doi:10.15620/cdc:108816

56. McIntyre A, Shepard M. Automatic insurance policies—important tools for preventing coverage loss. *N Engl J Med.* 2022;386(5):408-411. doi:10.1056/NEJMp2114189

57. Kaiser Family Foundation. Health coverage of immigrants. Published April 6, 2022. https://www.kff.org/racial-equity-and-health-policy/fact-sheet/health-coverage-of-immigrants/

58. Tolbert J, Orgera K, Damico A. Key facts about the uninsured population." *Kaiser Family Foundation.* Published November 6, 2020. https://www.kff.org/uninsured/issue-brief/key-facts-about-the-uninsured-population/

59. Coughlin T, Samuel-Jakubos H, Garfield R. Sources of payment for uncompensated care for the uninsured. *Kaiser Family Foundation.* Published April 6, 2021. https://www.kff.org/uninsured/issue-brief/sources-of-payment-for-uncompensated-care-for-the-uninsured/

Health Care Economics and Financing

Questions as you read through the chapter:

1. Health care costs a lot of money. What should we be spending that money on? What kinds of activities or goods should be reimbursed?
2. How is your clinician being paid? What are their incentives (or the incentives imposed upon them)?
3. How might switching to an alternative payment model change a clinician's incentives and day-to-day work?
4. How does the complexity of the system affect overall costs? How does the profit motive affect costs across the system?
5. How are prices determined? How *should* they be determined?

If you want to understand the health care system, it's essential to understand health economics and reimbursement—but being essential doesn't mean it's easy. We know these topics can be confusing and convoluted, as does anyone who's tried to purchase health insurance or understand why health care costs so dang much. We've done our best to reduce the abstractions and confusion, because the economics of health care is fascinating. Once you get the concepts down, you'll see how patients' and providers' behavior that seems to have nothing to do with money ends up affecting the bottom line and how the structure of the U.S. health care system influences that behavior. As the old joke goes, "The answer is money. Sorry, what was the question?"

Everything about health care discussed in Chapter 1 costs money, and money changes options, affects behavior, and creates problems. Insurance reimbursement—the way we pay for care—and economics—the study of the production, distribution, and consumption of that care—help to piece together what the problems are, what causes them, and how to fix them.

The Big Picture

How Much Does U.S. Health Care Cost?

In 2020, national health expenditures reached $4.1 trillion, which is $12,530 per person and 19.7% of the nation's GDP, far more than any other developed country.[1] In fact, the amount we in the United States spend on health care is larger than the *entire* economy of every country except China and Japan.[2] Spending varies widely by state, with Alaska spending nearly twice as much per capita as Utah.[3]

Given that share of GDP, the hospital and physician sectors are some of the largest in the entire U.S. economy. Compare to agriculture (0.8% of GDP) or arts and entertainment (1.1%).[4]

Where Does That $4.1 Trillion Come From and Where Does It Go?

To answer this question, let's look at two graphics.

First, Figure 3.1 is a simplified visual of the flow of funds, created by health economist Uwe Reinhardt. Although the $4.1 trillion spent annually

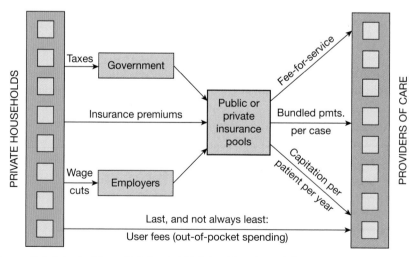

Who Pays for Health Care, and How Is It Paid?

Figure 3.1 Adapted from Reinhardt UE. *Priced Out*. 1st ed. Princeton University Press; 2019

on health care flows in incredibly complex and confusing pathways, this graphic gives a bird's-eye view of what the system looks like. Reinhardt also makes the point that, ultimately, all that money comes from individuals like you and me. (So whenever you read about government or employer contributions, remember that their funding comes from us, too.)

Next, Figure 3.2 is a more detailed breakdown of where the money comes from and where it goes. The first dollar bill shows the breakdown in health spending from public and private payers. The second dollar bill shows the portion of spending on medical care. We see that the plurality goes to hospitals.[a]

How Is That Spending Distributed Through the Population?

Spending is not spread evenly among all individuals. In fact, very few people account for the bulk of health spending—nearly half of health care spending was spent on just 5% of patients.[5] That's roughly three million people in the United States who each incurred an average of $127,284 a year on health-related expenses (see Section "Population Health and Delivery Innovations" in Chapter 1). In contrast, the bottom 50% of spenders (30% of whom are children) accounted for only 3.2% of spending.

How Are Costs Trending Over Time?

Health care spending has become a bigger and bigger portion of the GDP in the past 50 years. Health care spending grew faster than the economy for many years, and that growth hurt. As Jonathan Cohn puts it, "when national health care spending rises much more quickly than the economy is growing, you feel the impact—as relatively higher insurance premiums, higher out-of-pocket costs, and higher taxes to support government insurance programs."[6] For several years, though, the rate at which health spending outpaced the economy has been slowing. That is, overall spending is still growing; it just hasn't been accelerating as fast as it was before (Figure 3.3).

There were fears that the ACA (passed in 2010) might further accelerate costs, but as you can see from these graphs, that fear did not come to pass.[7] CMS tracks national health expenditures and makes predictions about the future of spending. CMS predicts that, by 2028, health spending will reach $6.2 trillion, still having grown faster than the rest of the economy.

You can find a million reports showing an uptrending growth line in health spending: spending goes up but doesn't come down. The one real exception comes in 2020, when the COVID-19 pandemic sharply—but

---

[a]For a beautiful visual display of all health expenditures—too big and complex to fit in this book—please see https://www.goinvo.com/vision/healthcare-dollars/.

Health Care Dollar

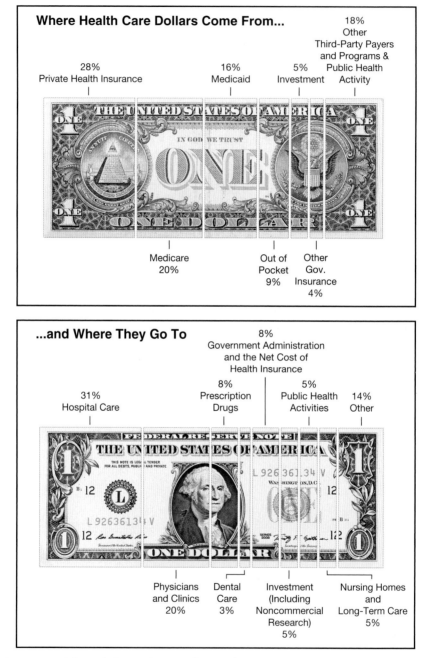

Where Health Care Dollars Come From...

18%
Other
Third-Party Payers
and Programs &
28%   16%   5%   Public Health
Private Health Insurance   Medicaid   Investment   Activity

Medicare
20%

Out of Pocket
9%

Other
Gov.
Insurance
4%

...and Where They Go To

8%
Government Administration
and the Net Cost of
Health Insurance

31%   8%   5%   14%
Hospital Care   Prescription   Public Health   Other
Drugs   Activities

Physicians
and Clinics
20%

Dental
Care
3%

Investment
(Including
Noncommercial
Research)
5%

Nursing Homes
and
Long-Term Care
5%

Figure 3.2 Adapted from Centers for Medicare & Medicaid Services. National Health Expenditure Fact Sheet, 2020. Accessed July 9, 2022. https://www.cms.gov/Research-Statistics-Data-and-Systems/Statistics-Trends-and-Reports/NationalHealthExpendData/NHE-Fact-Sheet

Average Annual Growth Rate of GDP per Capita and Total National Health Spending per Capita, by Decade

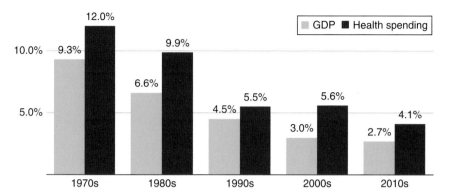

Figure 3.3 Adapted from Kurani N, Wager E, Amim K. How has U.S. spending on healthcare changed over time? Peterson-KFF Health System Tracker. Published February 25, 2022. https://www.healthsystemtracker.org/chart-collection/u-s-spending-healthcare-changed-time/#:~:text=From%201970%20through%201980%2C%20the,smaller%20margins%20in%20recent%20years

temporarily—decreased health spending,[b] during the initial suspension of nonemergency procedures, clinics canceling appointments, and patients postponing care because of fear of entering medical facilities.

Health Economics Concepts

Now you know the basics: health care costs $4.1 trillion, the bulk of that spending comes from public insurance and goes to hospitals, a very small number of people drive the bulk of spending, and spending is rising but no longer accelerating. Let's turn toward health economics concepts to help us understand a bit more. A health economist cares about the big picture: how do the "players" relate to each other, how does information flow (or not flow) among them, what kind of behaviors cause trends that might affect other aspects of the economic system? Consider the following concepts:

Information Asymmetry

Sometimes, one side of a transaction has more information than the other side. This is often the case for patients and providers, or patients and payers (ie, insurance plans). It often involves situations in which one side wants the other side to act on its behalf. One example of this would be a gastroenterologist who recommends getting a colonoscopy every 3 years—but the patient

---

[b]The decreased spending doesn't take into account the infusion of money from the federal government to help support hospitals and health facilities.

doesn't know that this recommendation goes against the guidelines or that the gastroenterologist owns the colonoscopy center. Another example is that, until recently, some contracts prohibited pharmacists from alerting patients that paying out of pocket for a medication would cost less than their copay through insurance.[8] (Luckily, this particularly egregious practice is now outlawed.[8])

Of course, it's neither fair nor efficient for one side of a transaction to know more about what's going on than the other does. Yet this happens all the time in health care.

Moral Hazard

Let's say you fall in love with a house on the beach, but it happens to sit on a stretch of the coast known for getting beaten in hurricane after hurricane. "That's too bad," you think, "but I guess insurance would pay for it," and you buy it anyway. That's moral hazard: the trend toward certain (usually more costly) behaviors when you know you won't end up having to cover the full cost.

In most cases human psychology is a little more complicated than that (a smoker doesn't keep smoking just because they know insurance would pay for any future lung cancer treatment, for instance), but moral hazard can drive low-value care, such as unnecessary magnetic resonance imaging (MRI) for routine low back pain, when patients don't have to pay the cost. Many think that moral hazard plays a big role in rising health care costs, and they feel that cost-sharing reduces its effects by making patients pay for some portion of the care they receive (this is what people refer to as "skin in the game").[c]

Adverse Selection

Insurance exists to spread costs among all beneficiaries in the pool, even those who don't end up needing any care. Yet, between a healthy 27-year-old versus a 55-year-old with diabetes who had a heart attack last year, who is more likely to purchase health insurance? If you're young and healthy, you might feel it's a good bet to risk not paying for health insurance at all. As costs of insurance go up, more and more people will make this same calculation and stop paying for insurance. Thus, the people left purchasing insurance will only be those who can expect to need more (and more expensive) care. The risk-spreading purpose of insurance is compromised, as the total number of people paying premiums goes down, whereas the amount of health spending stays high. That's adverse selection.

On the flip side, if a bunch of young, healthy people join the insurance pool, then the total number of people paying premiums goes up, whereas the health spending stays the same. This improves the risk-spreading purpose of

---

[c]There is surprisingly little research in this area, for how important it is to policy (see Section "Cost-Sharing" in Chapter 2).

insurance and lowers premiums. The individual mandate in the ACA was an attempt to harness that risk-spreading as a guard against adverse selection. After the mandate was made into a tax (by the Supreme Court in 2012) and then zeroed out (by the Trump administration in 2018), there were fears that instead adverse selection would lead to a "death spiral."[d] Although this did end up happening in a few markets in some states, luckily there was no overall death spiral.

Cost Versus Charge Versus Reimbursement

These words seem similar but refer to different things. Let's say a patient sees her physician to get a skin biopsy of a mole. To be in a position to perform that skin biopsy, the physician's office has to spend money, to pay rent, keep the lights on, buy gloves, buy a needle, pay nurses' salaries, etc. That's the provider's *cost*.[e] Then, the physician's office requests payment from the patient or insurance for the biopsy; that's the *charge* (or *price*, *fee*, or *bill*). Finally, the payer gives a certain amount to the physician's office for the biopsy; that's the *payment* or *reimbursement*.

In health care, the relationship between charge and cost is rarely clear. As the Robert Wood Johnson Foundation puts it:

> Little is known about how prices are derived. The answer to the basic question of what health care costs often is unknown. Payers see a bill, but generally are given very little detail about how prices in that bill are determined.[33]

To underscore this point, we can look at the fact that different payers reimburse different amounts for the same services. Keep this in mind when reading about health care costs and expenditures. Are we talking about the cost, the price (or charge or fee), or the amount reimbursed (the payment)? How would the difference matter in that situation? What is the true "cost" of a health care service, and how could we know this?

Rationing

Health care is a limited resource: there are restrictions on money, on providers, on time, on supplies, and on technology. Unless all world resources are devoted to health care, rationing must exist. And we already do it. That is a fact, so keep it in mind through every debate about rationing. The current

---

[d] A "death spiral" could ensue when the process of adverse selection ends up leaving only the highest cost patients purchasing insurance. Without any risk-spreading potential, the plan goes bankrupt, and no other insurance plans enter the market.

[e] Note that we sometimes use "cost" in this book to refer to the patient's cost, too, which is also entirely different, but the same word is used.

U.S. system rations by restricting access largely based on ability to pay. As the ethicist Peter Singer notes, for every patient we hear about in Britain who has to wait 3 months for a hip replacement or cannot get an experimental cancer treatment funded, there's an American who cannot afford a wheelchair or the standard-of-care cardiovascular medication.[9]

To understand health care, you must acknowledge and comprehend the ways that care is rationed and the effects of that rationing. All potential reform plans include rationing—even if they simply preserve the current practice. The real question is how to choose a method of rationing that is most equitable and sensible. Different ways to arrange a system of rationing may be:

By how much a given treatment will extend a patient's life or improve their quality of life[f] (eg, prioritize expensive, lifesaving measures for the young or otherwise healthy rather than for the elderly or very ill)

By a patient's ability to pay (eg, high deductibles for patients or low reimbursements for providers)

By first come, first served (eg, a waiting list)

By how well a treatment works compared to others (eg, prioritize treatments that have been proven to work well)

By prioritizing certain characteristics (eg, how sick patients are, or whether they are part of a high-priority group)

Which of these is most fair? Do some work better in some situations than in others? How might the decision change when you have fewer resources (ie, an organ transplant program, a wartime hospital, an underfunded rural clinic, or the initial COVID-19 surge in New York City) than when you have many resources?

Health Care Is Not a Normal Market

Traditional market economic theories are useful—but limited—in trying to understand the health care system. This is because health is not a normal good, and health care is not a normal market.

Supreme Court Justice Antonin Scalia once compared purchasing health insurance to purchasing broccoli. But are health decisions really comparable to purchasing goods? In purchasing health care services (for instance, surgery to remove an inflamed gallbladder in your 75-year-old mother), many factors, some of them unpredictable, produce the total expenditure. How long will your mother be in the hospital? What other medical conditions does she

[f] A commonly used metric is the Quality-Adjusted Life Year (QALY), which adjusts years of life added by the quality of those years. For example, a year of perfect health would rank as 1 QALY as a baseline, while a year of blindness might be 0.5 QALYs.

have? Will she have a difficult recovery? What medications will she need, and for how long? What tests will be run, and how many? What price negotiations did your insurance have with this hospital as opposed to the one down the street? When you buy groceries, all of your spending is known in advance, but that's not the case with health care.

Further, even if you could know how much it would cost you ahead of time, would that change her or your choices? Would she decide not to have gallbladder surgery? Would she risk leaving for another hospital? If so, would you also want to know about quality measures for your hospital, surgeon, and nurses? (Good luck finding that data on the spot.) What trade-off between cost and quality would be acceptable to your family? And what if the services she turned down were preventive, so her costs increased in the long run?

Often, the most expensive medical decisions are made by people under time constraints, at a vulnerable and scary time in their lives. Few have the clinical knowledge, desire, time, and logistical know-how to navigate the cheapest options for optimizing their health. Is making decisions about health—for which you will later receive a bill—really the same as choosing not to buy broccoli this week?

In fact, the health care system differs from a normal market in many ways beyond this example. Here are a few further examples from multiple sources[64-66]:

- **Lack of Price Transparency:** It is very difficult—often impossible—for patients to know what their bill will be before they receive care.
- **Insurance as Insulation:** Insurance shields the full brunt of prices from consumers so there is less pressure (economically and politically) to address them.
- **Conflicting Interests:** Physicians may act as both an agent for the patient as well as an independent business owner (or, more broadly, as someone who profits from the care they provide).
- **Tax Subsidies:** The tax subsidies provided to employers and employees to purchase insurance distort the market (see Section "Employer-Sponsored Insurance" in Chapter 2).
- **Failure of Competition:** Patients' choice of insurance plan or that of providers is often significantly constrained, without an ability to see an apples-to-apples comparison, meaning for many people they don't truly compete as market goods.
- **Suppliers Are Either Legally or Morally Required to Provide Services:** EDs are required to provide care, local or federal government often provides care for those who can't afford it, and providers (including both clinicians and hospitals) are limited by professional and legal limitations from withholding care from those who need it.

Our health—and our health care—is subject to forces outside of our control. It's also an emotionally and psychologically laden subject. You can choose not to buy a pound of mushrooms. You can't choose not to have stomach cancer or not to get hit by a car, and you can't expect someone with a health issue to make choices based solely on money. Although market forces can be useful in understanding and forming a better health care system, they are only part of the picture.

Understanding Reimbursement

Let's move on from concepts and get down to brass tacks: how providers are paid. Looking back (see Figure 3.2), we see that the bulk—59%—goes toward reimbursing care providers (clinicians, hospitals, nursing facilities, physical therapists, etc) for their work. Understanding how that reimbursement happens is pretty important: it is the primary mechanism for influencing provider behavior, makes up the bulk of health policy, and the details make up a big part of the day-to-day life of clinicians.

There are two basic reimbursement models for hospitals and clinicians: fee-for-service (FFS) and alternative payment models (APMs). We're going to put things in simple terms here, and add a little complexity later.

1. **FFS:** Care providers get a payment from the payer for each task or service they provide the patient. The more they do, the more they get paid. This is the most common form of reimbursement.

2. **APM (Also Called Value-Based Payment[8]):** Care providers get paid an amount that is adjusted based on the quality of their care and the complexity of their patients. Typically, they are also incentivized to lower the total cost of care, sometimes by being put on the hook for those costs themselves. This is a smaller but growing type of reimbursement.

Any reimbursement model has pros and cons, and each creates incentives and influences provider behavior, even if only unconsciously. For instance, if you're getting paid a fee for each service you provide, then you have an incentive to increase how much you provide a service, or to focus on the types of services that get paid the most. (In addition, you're being paid by how *much* you do, not how *well* you did it or if you helped the patient.) On the other hand, if you are getting paid per patient (capitation), you have an incentive to reduce the number of services you provide, because you make more profit the less you spend. Think of paying an electrician per outlet—and ending up with 50 outlets per room. Contrast that with paying the electrician a flat fee per house—and ending up with a single outlet in the whole place.

---

[8]You'll also hear this called Value-Based "Care," but we find the term "payment" to be more accurate.

No system can be perfect, so the question is how to design a system of payment that produces the best health outcomes for the most patients. Typically, the discussion focuses on paying for *value*, defined as health outcomes achieved per health care dollar spent.[10] But even defining value is tricky, much less figuring out how to incentivize it without causing any negative unintended consequences. For instance, if the electrician in the previous paragraph instead got paid based on how much his handiwork lowered people's electricity bills, he might strategically choose only to work with folks who had high bills to begin with (and thus more room to improve) and avoid those with drafty, energy-inefficient homes.

The Importance of Medicare in Reimbursement

Medicare is the dominant force in determining how providers are paid. With Medicare covering 14% of the population and paying for 21% of all health care spending, it is the nation's largest purchaser of services. Most providers cannot afford to lose out on that business, so they follow Medicare reimbursement rules closely. What's more, Medicaid and private insurance payers tend to base their own FFS reimbursement mechanisms on that of Medicare.

Medicare has also completely set the stage for APMs and value-based payments. Medicare is trying to transition all of their reimbursement from FFS to some form of an APM in the next 10 years, and private plans are making some movements toward value-based payments, as well.

For simplicity's sake, then, we will focus primarily on how Medicare handles both FFS and APM reimbursement. We'll walk through both of these categories of reimbursement for clinicians and hospitals, only skipping over a thing or two,[h] and then we'll end with a short word on reimbursement for postacute and home health care. Prescription drug reimbursement is discussed in Chapter 5.

Fee-for-Service

Even something seemingly simple, like getting paid a fee for something you do, is remarkably complex (notice a theme in this book?). We won't get into every detail here but will give a general understanding of key points.

What Is Being Paid for, and Why?

All medical services are assigned a code. The classification system for those codes, standardized for data gathering and billing, is called the Current Procedural Terminology (CPT). CPT was created in the 1960s by the American

---

[h]Just kidding! We simplify a lot. There's a reason health systems employ entire departments for this stuff.

Medical Association (AMA), and today, CPT codes are used by insurance plans for any diagnostic or therapeutic service a clinician can order or perform (ie, an x-ray, an office visit, a thyroid biopsy, earwax removal, alcohol misuse counseling, a cortisone injection into the shoulder, etc). Thus, CPT determines what is being paid for—the "service" in "FFS." The AMA still updates the CPT books annually, generating an annual revenue of $72 million (nearly double what they made in membership fees).[11]

CPT gives the "what" you are paying for—but payers still want to know the "why." So all CPT codes get associated with a diagnosis code. In order to standardize diagnosis naming for mortality statistics, the International Classification of Diseases (ICD) was formed around the turn of the 20th century. Over time, the diseases, symptoms, and injuries classified have grown exponentially, with the latest version, ICD-10, including 100,000 diagnoses.[i] In the United States, ICD-10 is also used to justify payment (ie, why you are providing the service), and most payers will deny payment for services unless they are associated with certain ICD-10 diagnoses. (Woe to the patient whose clinician codes "Z13.82 Screening for osteoporosis" to justify a bone density scan: Medicare won't pay for it unless she codes "Z78.0 Asymptomatic Menopausal State"!)

Sometimes clinicians select CPT and ICD-10 codes themselves to send on their bill to the payer. Many others, though, simply document their encounter in a note, and professional coders then "translate" this documentation into codes.

Who Is Being Paid?

FFS payments generally go to hospitals or to clinicians. Let's talk first about hospitals. Hospitals are paid for either *inpatient* or *outpatient* services.

The key concept to know about *inpatient hospital reimbursement* is the diagnosis-related group (DRG). DRGs are a classification system of how medically complex patients are and thus how much spending to expect them to have at the hospital.[j] To put it very simply, DRGs take into account the type of admitting diagnosis, severity of condition, whether a procedure took place, and the other medical conditions ("comorbidities") affecting or complicating care. One example is the DRG for an acute myocardial infarction ("heart attack"): without any complications, the average payment is $4,274.25, and with complications it is $9,580.68.[12]

DRGs have been used by Medicare since the 1980s as an attempt to rein in hospital spending. DRGs transition reimbursement from a *retrospective* (ie,

---

[i]The ICD-10 is frequently mocked for its hyper-specificity, like V97.33XD: Sucked into jet engine, subsequent encounter, or T63.442A: Toxic effect of venom of bees, intentional self-harm, initial encounter.
[j]Medicare does make allowances for cases that are unusually complicated and expensive. These "outlier cases" are billed separately and at a higher reimbursement rate than a typical DRG.

here's what I did, pay up) to a *prospective* (ie, here's how much a hospitalization should cost for someone this complex, so that's what we'll pay) payment system. Although other insurers can determine fees by other mechanisms (including paying per day in the hospital), most use the same or similar DRG system.

The DRG payment system has had a huge influence on providers and hospitals, including a significant reduction in average hospital length of stay for patients.[k] However, it may also drive what many consider too much focus on documenting irrelevant medical conditions or making conditions sound worse than they really are to make patients seem more complex—a phenomenon known as "upcoding"—rather than reducing unnecessary spending. Health information technology and EHRs have made it much easier to take a systematic and strategic approach to billing higher, and some hospitals have gotten in legal trouble for approaches that veered into fraud. For example, in 2020, Stanford Health Care was sued by the Department of Justice for their systematic coding practices.[13]

In contrast, the key concept to know about *clinician reimbursement* is the relative value unit (RVU).[l] Again, here Medicare sets the stage, releasing their Physician Fee Schedule every year. The relative value scale takes into account practice overhead and malpractice insurance costs, but about 50% of the RVU is due to how much "work" any service creates for a clinician (the "work" RVU or wRVU), so that each service can be compared to each other.

For example:

- a 30-minute office visit with a physician is 1.92 wRVUs,
- a screening colonoscopy is 3.26 wRVUs,
- admitting a complex patient to the hospital is 3.86 wRVUs,
- surgery to replace a hip joint is 19.6 wRVUs.

RVUs are recommended by the AMA committee and usually approved by CMS. The process by which RVUs are determined is controversial, and many feel that it overly values doing procedures in comparison to thinking about or talking to patients (see Section "Setting Payments to Physicians, Part 1: the RVU Update Committee" in Chapter 6). In 2021, Medicare took this

---

[k]This shift to shorter hospital stays has pros and cons. Though many patients may be glad not to spend the night in a hospital, discharging patients before they're ready has negative consequences both for health (due to incomplete care) as well as for costs (through readmissions and avoidable health outcomes). On the other hand, keeping patients in the hospital for too long puts them at increased risk for hospital-acquired infections and medical errors, and each extra day in the hospital can cost $10,000 or more.

[l]Reimbursement for advanced practice providers (nurse practitioners and physician assistants) is a little more complicated and usually set lower than what a physician gets.

criticism to heart, shifting some RVUs higher for "cognitive" work as opposed to "procedure" work.

Each year, Medicare then sets the amount they pay per RVU, called a conversion factor. This usually goes up over time but can go down—as it did in 2021, keeping the overall level of payment the same even as RVUs went up.

Remember, although DRGs and RVUs determine payment for services, they do not constrain how frequently those services get rendered.[m] Medicare expenditures do in fact vary a lot around the country, but that variation is in *volume* of a service, not in payment per service. The Dartmouth Atlas tracks these variations with interactive maps you can view online (Figure 3.4). Reimbursements are price adjusted and include parts A and B.

Reimbursements per Medicare Enrollee, by Region, 2018

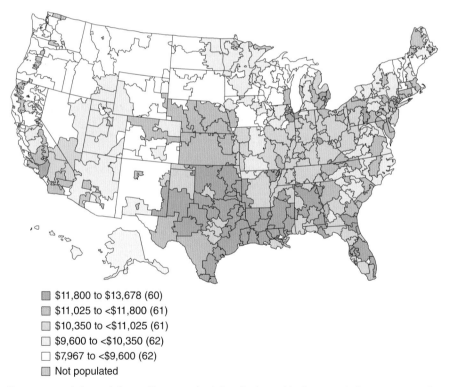

- ■ $11,800 to $13,678 (60)
- ■ $11,025 to <$11,800 (61)
- ■ $10,350 to <$11,025 (61)
- ☐ $9,600 to <$10,350 (62)
- ☐ $7,967 to <$9,600 (62)
- ■ Not populated

Figure 3.4 Adapted from Dartmouth Atlas Project. Medicare reimbursements—by HRR. 2019. https://www.dartmouthatlas.org/interactive-apps/medicare-reimbursements/#hrr

---

[m]With some exceptions, like global surgery periods.

Here is where Medicare differs from other plans. Whereas most insurance payers have to negotiate rates and reimbursement amounts with various providers, Medicare instead publishes a standard fee schedule for providers to take it or leave it. They generally take it.

Again, Medicare dominates the reimbursement landscape here. Many plans negotiate their rates as a percent of Medicare payments (private insurance usually higher than Medicare,[n] and Medicaid always less), and the annual Medicare fee schedule is closely watched by clinicians and health systems nationwide.

Because Medicare has a set fee schedule, they may reimburse less than what a hospital claims that their services actually cost them. See Figure 3.5,

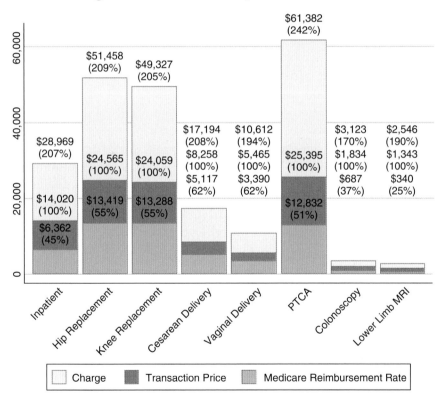

Charges and Reimbursement, Selected Procedures

Figure 3.5 MRI, magnetic resonance imaging ; PTCA, percutaneous transluminal coronary angioplasty Adapted from Cooper Z, Craig SV, Gaynor M, Reenen JV. The price ain't right? hospital prices and health spending on the privately insured*. *Q J Econ.* 2019;134(1):51-107. doi:10.1093/qje/qjy020

---

[n]On average, private insurers reimburse at about 250% of Medicare rates. https://www.rand.org/pubs/research_reports/RR3033.html

in which the amount Medicare pays ("Medicare reimbursement rate") is much lower than the negotiated rates that private insurance pays ("Transaction price"), which are themselves much lower than what hospitals list as the charge ("charge price").

For a long time, there was controversy around something called "cost shifting," a theory that, when Medicare set reimbursements too low, hospitals and systems merely shifted those costs to higher fees from private insurance. This, however, has been debunked from both liberal and conservative economists.[14] As well-known conservative health economist Avik Roy tweeted, "Way back when, I used to subscribe to the cost-shifting thesis. But the overwhelming evidence is that hospitals make up their cost figures, and charge higher prices to the privately insured because they can."[15,o]

Variation in FFS Payments by Private Insurers

Private insurers negotiate with providers to set their fees. This leads to enormous variation in reimbursement amounts, in multiple domains:

■ A hospital can get reimbursed different amounts for the same service by different payers.

■ A payer can pay different amounts for the same service at different hospitals in the same city.

■ A payer can pay different amounts for the same service at the same hospital, based on different plans (ie, preferred provider organization [PPO] vs point of service [POS]; most insurance companies have a multitude of different plans, which may separately negotiate their own reimbursement rates).

This process has led to some truly wild variation in terms of how much services are reimbursed. A substantial amount of research has been done on this variation, frequently focused on joint replacements (Figure 3.6) and MRIs.

Keep in mind, of course, that these hospitals may publish a different price for this service altogether, in their "charge master." (Remember, charge—or price—does not equal reimbursement.) In 2021, the federal government began requiring hospitals to publicly publish the complete list of prices they negotiate with insurers. The *New York Times* published some of these, including the fact that a colonoscopy at the University of Mississippi Medical Center costs $1,463 with a Cigna plan versus $2,144 with an Aetna plan versus $782 if you pay out of pocket.[16]

°Note that Roy is using "charge" and "price" a little loosely here. Technically, hospitals make up their charges, and then they negotiate higher reimbursement rates because they can.

Average Charges for Hip and Knee Replacements in Large Employer Plans, by Region, 2018

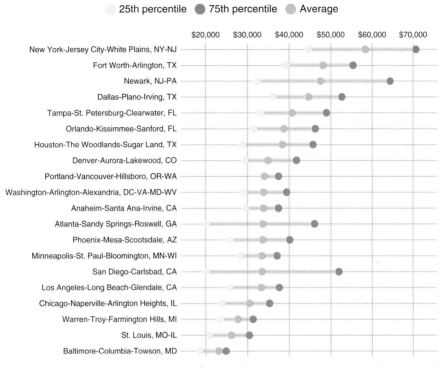

Figure 3.6 Note: Results shown for 20 largest MSAs, by population, with available data. (Adapted from Kurani N, Rae M, Pollitz K, et al. Price transparency and variation in U.S. health services. Peterson-KFF Health System Tracker. Published January 13, 2021. https://www.healthsystemtracker.org/brief/price-transparency-and-variation-in-u-s-health-services/)

To quote health economist Uwe Reinhardt: "In a nutshell, chaos reigns."[17]

APMs and Value-Based Payment

This section connects and cross-references to a lot of other sections in this book, including population health in Chapter 1, Medicare Advantage (MA) in Chapter 2, choosing the right metrics in Chapter 4, and Quality Payment Program and CMMI in Chapter 6. We won't repeat all of that information here, so we'll ask that you check those sections out to fully engage with this one.

APM refers to any reimbursement system that isn't just FFS, and which almost always incorporates value-based payments (ie, payment based on meeting quality metrics). APMs and value-based payments have really taken

Table 3.1   But What *Is* an APM? APMs Fall Into One of Three Basic Categories of APMs

1	FFS payments + bonus payments based on quality metrics	Typically paid to providers Example: Pay for Performance 19.8% of total provider reimbursement in 2020
2	FFS payments + accountability for total health spending of beneficiaries (ie, "risk") + adjustment for quality metrics	Typically paid to providers that have chosen to "take on risk" together, sometimes as a foray into APMs even while still participating in FFS Example: Accountable Care Organization 34.2% of total provider reimbursement in 2020
3	Population-based payments (ie, "risk") + adjustment for quality metrics	Typically paid to providers experienced in APMs who are totally committed to "taking on risk" together Example: Primary Care First 6.2% of total provider reimbursement in 2020

Source: Adapted from HCPlan. *APM Measurement: Progress of Alternative Payment Models.* 2021. http://hcplan.org/workproducts/APM-Methodology-2020-2021.pdf

off since 2010, but FFS remains the dominant form of reimbursement. Even within APMs, FFS payments are common, as many APMs only add bonuses and penalties on top of an FFS foundation. By 2020, although 60% of all health care dollars in the United States was paid through some form of an APM, only 6.2% of reimbursement was through an APM that did not use any component of FFS. Although Medicare is best known for piloting APMs, even private payers make nearly half of their reimbursement payments through one[18] (Table 3.1).

But What Is an APM?

There's quite a bit of variation and nuance in APMs, but a couple of key concepts tend to hold them together. First, all APMs incorporate quality metrics as part of reimbursement. There are many, many (many) quality metrics, with examples being things like ensuring patients get a medication reconciliation postdischarge from a hospital (see Chapter 4), or how many patients have well-controlled blood pressure. Generally, providers can pick and choose which metrics they get graded on.

Second, most APMs incentivize keeping costs down. The incentive is usually through "taking on risk,"[p] that is, being held accountable for the total health spending of your patient population. To do this, it is necessary to develop spending targets—ie, how much *should* a group of patients cost—with bonuses or penalties depending on whether your patient population ends up under- or overshooting that target. Risk can be "upside" or "1 sided" (ie, you benefit if you undershoot but are not penalized if you overshoot) or it can be "downside" or "2 sided" (ie, you benefit if you undershoot and you are penalized if you overshoot).

But wait … if you incentivize a health system to lower their patients' health spending (to undershoot the target), couldn't they just lower costs by refusing to care for the sickest patients? That's what happened under managed care in the 1990s.[19] Using the average cost to determine spending targets actually incentivizes APMs to seek out the healthiest patients and try to avoid caring for the sickest (this is called cherry-picking). Because, although average Medicare[q] spending per beneficiary is $11,523 per year,[20] that average hides a lot of variation: some patients cost next to nothing, and some sicker patients cost millions.

That's where *risk-adjustment* comes in, an absolutely essential element of APMs. If you're trying to move payments from volume to value, then you need to have an idea of how much a patient population should cost, so you can determine cost targets and savings. Some hospitals and some insurance plans spend more on their patients because the group they care for really *is* sicker. So, many APMs are "*risk adjusted*," meaning that payments are higher for patient populations who have more—and more serious—medical conditions.[r]

Understanding how risk-adjustment affects spending targets is essential to understanding how APMs operate. Imagine you are a provider in an APM. Here's a simplified explanation of how your spending target—and savings or losses—gets developed:

1. When clinicians see patients throughout the year, they document every medical condition that the patient has.
2. The clinician or coder sends ICD-10 codes for those conditions[s] on a bill to the payer.

---

[p]Another way of putting this is that Medicare is putting providers' "skin in the game," like patients and cost-sharing (see Section "Cost-Sharing" in Chapter 2).

[q]Traditional Medicare (ie, those in Part A), not MA. For MA, the average payments were $11,844 per beneficiary.

[r]Interestingly, this further entrenches ICD-10 diagnosis coding even as it lessens the importance of RVUs and DRGs.

[s]These are called "hierarchical condition categories," or HCCs.

3. The payer converts each code to a numerical score and adds them up. For instance, diabetes without complication (0.105) plus depression (0.343) plus pneumonia (0.131) = 0.579.

4. Do steps 1 to 3 for every patient in your population, then average the scores for all of your patients together to get your "risk adjustment factor."[t]

5. Multiply your risk-adjustment factor by the nationwide average of expected patient spending, and then multiply that by the size of your population to get your target spending (ie, "benchmark").

6. At the end of the year, compare your population's actual spending to your target. Did they spend less? Great! You get to keep some or all of the savings. Did they spend more? Boo! You have to cut a big check to the payer for some or all of that extra cost.

Because of how an accounting of medical conditions ends up affecting the target spending, you can imagine that providers in APMs expend a lot of energy on ensuring a complete list of the "right" diagnosis codes gets sent for every patient. The same concerns about upcoding exist here, as with DRGs, particularly as more and more plans take part in risk-adjustment over time.

There are many examples of APMs, too many to review here. However, we do want to talk about two important examples here, because you're sure to hear about them: accountable care organizations (ACOs) and MA.

Accountable Care Organizations (ACOs)

The most widespread APM might be ACOs, which were popularized by the ACA and piloted by the CMMI. ACOs are an example of Category 2 from table 3.1. Since 2017, there have been about 1,000 ACOs,[21] which can contract with either public or private payers, and in total include over 32 million people.[22] And over 500 of those ACOs contract with Medicare, covering more than one-fifth of all Medicare patients.[23,24]

An ACO is not an insurance plan. Rather, ACOs are groups of providers (almost always includes primary care providers but often also includes hospitalists, specialists, home health, etc) who agree to take on the responsibility for costs and quality of a large group of patients, from 5,000 patients up to 250,000 or more. That large group of patients, called the ACO's population, gets assigned to the ACO through complex rules depending on the payer. Although the ACO likely offers certain extra services to the patients—like transportation, home visits, and nurse visits that would never be reimbursed under traditional FFS payments—very likely those patients won't have any idea they are part of an ACO.

---

[t]To help prevent gaming the system, these scores are normalized across the nation, with the average score being set at "1."

The ACO providers still get paid for their services (so they haven't left FFS altogether), but they have a competing interest to constrain that spending below the benchmark. If their population spends less than the benchmark, then the ACO gets to split the savings with the payer (ie, "shared savings"); if the population spends more than the benchmark, the ACO may have to pay a penalty. For instance, in 2020, Medicare ACOs saved Medicare $4.1 billion, of which $2.3 billion was sent to ACOs as a shared savings bonus. The ACO also has to meet a list of quality metrics, to show that they aren't just reducing spending at the expense of quality. In 2020, 97% of Medicare ACOs met the quality metrics defined by CMS.

Not all of the evidence is so rosy, though. ACOs seem to gain initial savings early on and then even out,[25] and they also are most efficient when forced to take on downside risk[26]—which can be a very hard change to make. You can imagine how difficulties might arise in a health system—like an ACO that includes both clinicians and a hospital—that still relies on revenue from those expensive hospital services they are supposed to be reducing. Any health system contracts with many different payers, and having both an ACO population as well as an FFS population means a health system is operating in two diametrically opposed business models at the same time. It's a little like entrusting bartenders and bar owners to decrease alcohol spending.

Medicare Advantage (MA)

MA adds a whole other layer of complexity to understanding APMs. MA plans are private companies—usually large insurers such as UnitedHealth or Aetna—which contract with CMS to handle the spending for a population of Medicare patients. Unlike ACOs, patients are not assigned; rather, the MA plans advertise and entice people to sign up. The population in an MA plan goes through a similar benchmarking process as that of ACOs to determine how much their entire population of patients should cost. Then, CMS pays a flat fee based on that benchmark per member per month (ie, capitation or population-based payment) to the MA plan. In contrast to FFS, where providers get paid more and more for doing more and more, under capitation MA plans get paid the same amount[u] no matter what their patient population's actual health expenditures are.

MA plans, having contracted with CMS, now have to turn around and contract with providers, the same as any private insurance plan discussed in Chapter 2 (an MA plan can be a health maintenance organization [HMO], a PPO, etc). Although MA plans often offer improved benefits[v] compared to traditional Medicare, they also may engage in more utilization management

---

[u]Subject, of course, to quality metrics and the medical loss ratio (see Chapter 2).
[v]Better benefits from MA plans include things like transportation, dental, vision, and hearing coverage.

tactics (see Chapter 2), such as narrow networks. Interestingly, although MA is paid in population-based payments by CMS, about 40% of how they in turn reimburse providers is through traditional FFS (without quality bonuses or shared savings).

MA plans, as middlemen, make money by spending less on care than they have received from CMS. In order to do this, MA plans need to either (a) increase their benchmarking and payments from CMS and/or (b) decrease patients' spending.[w] It turns out that it's easiest to increase the benchmarking through risk-adjustment. Although ACOs benefit from risk-adjustment, MA plans are particularly known for more intensive practices, which have been called out by Medicare[27] and have even gotten some plans in trouble with the Department of Justice for fraud.[28,29] But intensive risk-adjustment continues because it works, with high margins, as shown in Figure 3.7.[30]

The initial idea behind CMS contracting with private insurance plans was to lower costs and improve choice—though it hasn't always turned out that way. On the whole, MA has not yet saved the government money. In fact,

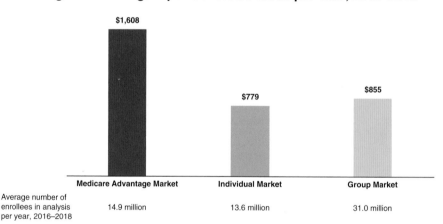

Average Gross Margins per Covered Person per Year, 2016–2018

	Medicare Advantage Market	Individual Market	Group Market
	$1,608	$779	$855
Average number of enrollees in analysis per year, 2016–2018	14.9 million	13.6 million	31.0 million

Figure 3.7 Note: The group market only includes fully insured plans. Enrollment numbers do not include plans that do not file data with the NAIC, plans licensed as life insurance. California health maintenance organizations regulated by California's Department of Managed Health Care; plans that recorded negative premiums, claims, or enrollment numbers; or plans domiciled outside of the United States. Figures are averaged across 2016, 2017, and 2018. (Adapted from https://www.kff.org/report-section/financial-performance-of-medicare-advantage-individual-and-group-health-insurance-markets-issue-brief/)

---

[w]They can also affect payments by improving their quality—called "star" ratings—but we won't get into the weeds on that here.

CMS pays an average of 4% more per capita for MA beneficiaries than they do for similar patients in traditional Medicare.[31]

It's complicated and controversial. Some studies do indicate cost savings for MA plans, some show improved utilization of health care services,[32] and some show improved quality. There is heated debate on whether MA is a scam on taxpayers, a promising program in need of reform, or a godsend.[x] Regardless, considering 48% of all Medicare beneficiaries are now covered by an MA plan, it's clear that MA—and thus the privatization of Medicare—is more than just a trend.

Reimbursement for All Other Care Services

We've talked a lot about Medicare and how it reimburses hospitals and clinicians—now let's take a peek at how everyone else gets reimbursed. Even though hospital and clinician services make up the bulk of reimbursement, there's still a lot of other care to be paid for. This category includes a huge variety of types of services with many different rules for each: postacute care, home health, long-term support services, medical equipment, lab services, ambulance services, etc. We won't go into all the details here, but let's at least talk about postacute and long-term care in nursing facilities, most of which is paid for by public insurance.

Medicare will pay for short-term stays in postacute care facilities (ie, skilled nursing facilities [SNFs], see Chapter 1). To qualify, the patient must have spent at least three nights[y] in a hospital, and either physical or occupational therapy must be the primary reason for postacute care. Postacute care facilities get paid a daily rate (determined by a complicated formula, of course). The daily rate goes down as the stay extends; patients have a copay after day 21, and Medicare won't pay at all after day 100 for a spell of illness. Daily rates for an urban SNF average $434.95, and SNF spending totaled $27.8 billion in 2019.[33]

Although Medicare doesn't pay for long-term care in nursing homes, Medicaid does, with a daily rate called a per diem. The details of setting that per diem vary widely by state, but a rough idea is around $200; note this is much lower than the payment for postacute care. All the same, spending on long-term support services—nearly all of which goes to nursing facilities—represents about one-third of all Medicaid spending.[34]

---

[x]For a good summary of this debate see the MA point–counterpoint articles in Health Affairs recommended in Suggested Reading.
[y]This requirement was waived during the public health emergency rules of the COVID-19 pandemic, and for many ACOs on a long-term basis.

The (Big) Business of Medicine

Now is a good time to switch gears. You've read through how health care providers—ie, hospitals, health systems, clinics, and clinicians—get reimbursed. Those providers are also businesses. A century ago, most "business" of medicine was the doctor himself, who accepted payments directly from his patients—who were part of his community—for his services. Not so today: health care is Big Business.

There are various ways to think about the strength of a business, and you can find quite different numbers from different sources. In Table 3.2, we show one lens, which is return on capital (or the ratio of earnings to investment). Note this is different from profits: a pharmaceutical company is vastly more profitable than a pharmacy—but the pharmaceutical company has to invest more capital into making their business run. Although there's also a lot of variance within each of these groups, we see that the businesses that are most transactional (ie, buy from one place and sell to another) also have the best return on capital.[z]

As much as we emphasized how health care is different from normal markets, the question of how to make money in medicine does align with the normal business world. One strategy is to consolidate market power. Another

Table 3.2 Health Industry: Return on Capital in 2017

Pharmacies	18%
Drug wholesalers	15%
Pharmacy benefits managers (PBMs)	12%
Health insurance plans	12%
Pharma companies	11%
Device/tech companies	10%
Hospitals in a network/system	7%
Independent hospitals	4.5%

Source: Adapted from Leste T, Siegel Y, Shukla M. Return on capital performance in life sciences and health care. https://www2.deloitte.com/content/dam/Deloitte/ec/Documents/life-sciences-health-care/DI_Investment-view-of-health-care-market.pdf; Consolidation in California's health care market 2010-2016: impact on prices and ACA premiums. Nicholas C. Petris Center on Health Care Markets and Consumer Welfare. School of Public Health. University of California, Berkeley. Published March 26, 2018. http://petris.org/wp-content/uploads/2018/03/CA-Consolidation-Full-Report_03.26.18.pdf

[z]Note that you'll get different numbers from different sources. For simplicity and consistency, we went with numbers from a single source.

is to find an inefficiency in a business process and figure out how to improve it as a useful middleman (like those transactional businesses in the table). Both of these strategies are seen extensively in health care. Let's talk about consolidation first, as a general trend. Then we will talk about middlemen, focused on a single, but very powerful, example.

Networks and Consolidation

In the past, physicians were typically small business owners, either solo practitioners or part of a physician-run medical group. In the past decade, however, physicians have increasingly become employees, with older doctors selling their practices and younger doctors not bothering with private practice at all. In California from 2010 to 2016, physicians working for hospital foundations increased from 24% to 39%, and for specialists it was up to 50%.[35] From 2016 to 2018, hospital systems bought 8,000 medical practices, and 14,000 physicians became hospital-affiliated employees.[36] As of 2018, more U.S. physicians are employees rather than owners of their own practices[37] (Figure 3.8).

Similarly, hospitals themselves have been merging and consolidating into networks. In 2016, research found that 90% of regions were highly consolidated for hospitals (ie, not much competition), up from 65% in 1990.[38] An example of this is Sutter Health, which owns 24 hospitals and 34 surgery centers

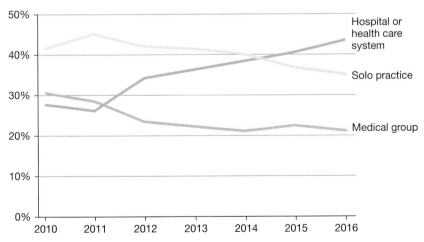

Percentages of Primary Care Physicians Working in Organizations, by Ownership Type, 2010-2016

Figure 3.8 Adapted from Fulton BD. Health care market concentration trends in the United States: evidence and policy responses. *Health Affairs*. Published September 2017. https://www.healthaffairs.org/doi/10.1377/hlthaff.2017.0556

in Northern California, employing thousands of physicians and boasting an operating revenue of $13 billion in 2018.[39]

Why does this matter? Health economists have found that consolidation generally leads to increased prices (even up to 20%!), because of increased bargaining power with insurers, without improving quality of care.[40] And price increase does appear to have happened where Sutter operates, in Northern California:

> In Northern California—which is considerably more concentrated than Southern California across all measures of health care market concentration that we analyzed—inpatient prices were 70% higher, outpatient prices were 17-55% higher (depending on the specialty of physician performing the procedure), and ACA premiums were 35% higher than they were in Southern California. Even after adjusting for input cost differences (i.e. wages) between Northern California and Southern California, procedure prices are still often 20-30% higher in Northern California than Southern California.[35]

In 2019, Sutter agreed to settle a lawsuit about this, which alleged that they used their consolidated market power to raise prices, that is, acting as a monopoly, for which they paid $575 million.[41] (Sutter still faces an ongoing federal antitrust lawsuit, as well.)

If we care about high prices in health care, then of course we should think hospital and health system consolidation matters. We also wonder what else these trends—particularly with the "employee-ization" of physicians—might tell us. Are physicians just suddenly less interested in running their own practice than they were 30 years ago? Or could this reflect intolerably high costs of the current landscape, that is, wanting to offload some of the expense of EHRs, reporting quality measures, and navigating incredibly complex reimbursement rules from a plethora of payers—not to mention negotiating power with payers—so they can just focus on providing care to their patients? Certainly, the decrease in revenue during the COVID-19 pandemic hit small and solo practices particularly hard, underscoring the strengthening of their business that consolidation might offer in weathering difficult periods.

And it's not just hospitals doing the consolidating, either. Another, more recent, trend is the purchase of medical practices, nursing homes, hospitals, and hospital networks by private equity groups. Private equity (ie, non-publicly traded investment firms) typically buy and restructure companies to make them more profitable. As of 2021, private equity firms own about 4% of hospitals, 11% of nursing homes, and 2% of MA plans[42]—but their greatest focus is on purchasing outpatient specialty practices.[43] There have been high-profile criticisms of private equity in health care, notably with the purchase and closure of Hahnemann Hospital in Philadelphia in 2018,[aa] which primarily served low-income and vulnerable patients. The overall research, however, has not yet pointed toward any clear trends in terms of cost or quality from private equity ownership.

Consolidation has become prevalent in other parts of the health care system, as well. For example, the largest employer of physicians in the United States is now an insurance company (UnitedHealth Care[44]), and the retail chain CVS owns both the large insurer Aetna as well as a major mail-order pharmacy and pharmacy benefits manager (PBM), Caremark.

Growth of Middlemen: Spotlight on PBMs

Middlemen abound in health care, but here we'll focus on just one prominent, important example. PBMs are companies that operate in the middle between pharmaceutical companies, pharmacies, and payers. PBMs manage prescription drug benefits for insurance plans, by negotiating prices and rebates with pharmaceutical companies, developing networks of acceptable pharmacies (similar to networks for providers), and using strategies to direct patients away from more expensive medications, called "drug utilization management" (see Section "Paying for Prescription Drugs" in Chapter 5). You may have never heard of a PBM or known that one was involved in your prescriptions, but PBMs serve nearly 270 million Americans (almost all of us!). Consolidation happens in this area, too, with the three largest PBMs—Express Scripts, CVS Caremark, and OptumRx—controlling 89% of the market.[45]

PBMs present themselves as lowering drug costs for payers and patients; for instance, the industry says it will save consumers $1 trillion in the 2020s.[46] However, others criticize PBMs for taking too big of a slice from the middle, see Figure 3.9, and for enlarging the size of the pie (ie, propping up the system of high prices).

First, PBMs receive rebates directly from drug companies, which totaled nearly $90 billion in 2016.[47] The practices around rebates are not transparent, and many payers complain that these are not passed on to them or their customers as savings; for their part, drug companies state these rebates necessitate raising prices even further. Second, PBMs sometimes take too large a cut from the payment between insurance plans and pharmacies, called "spread pricing." Third, PBMs used "gag orders" in their contracts to prevent pharmacists from telling patients when it would be cheaper to buy a medication out of pocket than to bill insurance—thankfully, this practice got outlawed in 2018.[8]

[aa]For more, read https://www.newyorker.com/magazine/2021/06/07/the-death-of-hahnemann-hospital

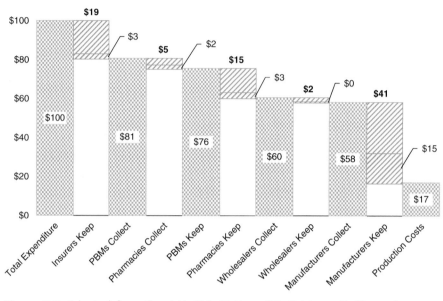

Figure 3.9 Adapted from Sood N, Shih T, Nuys KN, Goldman D. Flow of money through the pharmaceutical distribution system. USC Schaeffer. Published June 6, 2017. https://healthpolicy.usc.edu/research/flow-of-money-through-the-pharmaceutical-distribution-system/

Whether you think PBMs offer an overall useful service, it's hard to look at the flow of a hypothetical $100 spent on pharmaceuticals—which cost $17 to produce—in Figure 3.9 and claim that the process is efficient.

Why Does U.S. Health Care Cost So Much?

This question has a lot of answers, and you'll hear a different prioritization of and opinion on these answers depending on whom you talk to. When it comes down to it, health expenditures are made up of (a) price of services and (b) volume of services. Here, we will present 10 categories of factors that affect price and volume, and no answer about high expenditures is complete without addressing each. Let's go through them.

"It's the Prices, Stupid"

In 2003, health economist Uwe Reinhardt wrote a seminal article titled "It's the Prices, Stupid: Why the United States Is So Different From Other Countries." To quote from that paper's conclusion:

In 2000 the United States spent considerably more on health care than any other country, whether measured per capita or as a percentage of GDP. At the same time, most measures of aggregate utilization such as physician visits per capita and hospital days per capita were below the OECD median. Since spending is a product of both the goods and services used and their prices, this implies that much higher prices are paid in the United States than in other countries. But U.S. policymakers need to reflect on what Americans are getting for their greater health spending. They could conclude: It's the prices, stupid.

It's been 20 years since that article was published, but the data he presents (the ratio of U.S. health care spending to utilization is much higher than comparable countries) have only worsened over time.[48] At the most basic level, the answer to why U.S. health care costs so much is that we pay high prices for it (Figure 3.10)!

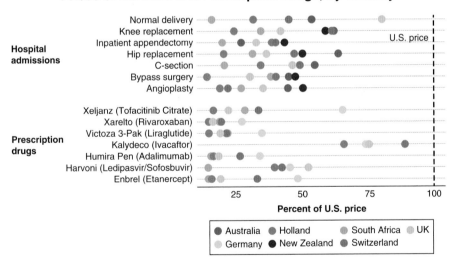

Prices of Services and Prescription Drugs, by Country

Figure 3.10 Note: Data are from International Federation of Health Plans member companies in eight countries. International service price comparisons are complicated by potentially different service definitions, reimbursement arrangements, and health plan participation across countries. (Adapted from Nunn R, Parsons J, Shambaugh J. A dozen facts about the economics of the US health-care system. Brookings. Published March 2020. https://www.brookings.edu/research/a-dozen-facts-about-the-economics-of-the-u-s-health-care-system/)

Lack of Transparency and Information Asymmetry

Insurers know what things cost because they negotiate (or, in the case of public insurance, set) their reimbursement rates. No such transparency exists for individual patients, though. Individuals are often asked to account for costs in their medical decision-making; however, many barriers stand in their way:

Hospitals, physicians, and insurance plans don't provide up-front information about comparative prices and billing.

Patients haven't had access to national data or average costs.

Even if patients could access the above data, they would need to compare costs at all regional hospitals and be willing to switch hospitals even if they are in critical condition.

Patients have no way of knowing whether *their own care* would be comparable to the cost estimates they might be given. (Their illness may be more severe, they may have more or fewer comorbidities, their care may have more or fewer complications, etc.)

Patients usually don't understand how medical billing works.

Patients usually don't have time to hassle with billing forms and learn about coverage rules.

Patients lack the clinical knowledge in comparing the added value of a more expensive treatment.

And we haven't even mentioned pharmaceuticals yet.

Not only is the above true for patients, in many cases it's also true for clinicians. The two people in the room making health care decisions—the clinician and the patient—may be those who have the least access to knowledge about what those decisions will cost.

Lack of Standardization and Coordination

The U.S. system is decentralized and there is no one standard for how anything gets done. Billing is a great example of how lack of centralization or standardization drives up costs. Each payer has its own (often quite extensive) rules about billing, and each provider has to learn and apply these. Each health care facility must pay for its own dedicated billing department or pay to outsource it (unlike, say, in England, where billing is a centralized organization). This billing workforce cost has played a role in the decreasing ability of physicians to maintain private practices.[ab]

[ab]Many offices and hospitals outsource their billing services to a specialized business, like the Medical Billing Service, and, as is a trend in other areas of health care, some of this outsourcing is going abroad in an attempt to reduce costs. Interestingly, privacy concerns have both increased billing needs (by increasing the amount of paperwork required by law) and constrained cost reduction (by raising concerns about privacy in outsourcing).

Sometimes it feels like as much or more energy is spent on figuring out how to bill medical care as on giving the care itself. In fact, in 2011, research found that "US nursing staff, including medical assistants, spent 20.6 hours per physician per week interacting with health plans," costing $82,975 per physician annually.[39] Although billing—and FFS—gets a bad rap here, it is also worth remembering that administrative burden may not be decreased in Value-Based Payment programs, which typically require quite a bit of documentation for quality metrics. Patients—and society— might fairly ask if the money on administrative complexity is well spent (Figure 3.11).

The level of decentralization also means inefficient coordination—if any at all—between different organizations providing different aspects of care. Only rarely are these connected to one another, and a patient may end up receiving care from multiple organizations without their working together. Let's review an example, which no one who works in health care will find unrealistic. Let's say Ms. M is admitted to Hospital X for a broken hip after getting hit by a car. She gets a computed tomography (CT) scan, which shows a small brain bleed. After surgical repair of her hip, she's discharged to SNF, but after a few days she becomes confused and is sent to

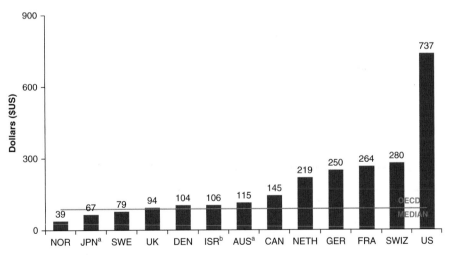

Spending on Health Insurance Administration per Capita, 2014

Figure 3.11 Adjusted for differences in cost of living. OECD, Organisation for Economic Co-operation and Development. [a]Data from 2013 in Australia, Japan. [b]Data from Israel. (Adapted from Commonwealth Fund. OECD health data 2016. https://www.commonwealthfund.org/sites/default/files/documents/___media_files_publications_chartbook_2016_att_fsarnak2016_oecd_data_chartpack_final_pdf.pdf)

the ED at Hospital Z. Hospital Z doesn't have access to her records from Hospital X, so they repeat much of the same blood tests and CT scan of her head. Eventually, she's discharged home with a home health agency, but the medications from her pharmacy don't match the med list from Hospital X or from Hospital Z, and she ends up taking too much blood pressure medication. No one has helped her get a timely appointment with her PCP, so she goes to an urgent care, where they don't have access to any of her records, she doesn't remember her brain bleed, and they prescribe aspirin. Ms. M's head bleed thus worsens and she gets confused again, so she's taken back to Hospital X, where they have no record of anything that happened since she was discharged the first time, and they get a third CT scan. These separate entities—two different hospitals, a nursing facility, pharmacy, doctor's office, urgent care, and home health agency—do not have any incentive to share information and efficiently coordinate Ms. M's care.[49] In this case, not only did the lack of coordination lead to frustrating and poor quality of care for Ms. M, it also led to wasteful spending (see the Case Study on Hospital Readmissions at the end of this book).

Lack of Governmental Regulation

Governments in Japan, Germany, and England (among others) strictly regulate payments in health care. For instance, in Japan, the government decides what physicians may charge for any service. In England, the government negotiates down the price of pharmaceuticals.

Certainly, Medicare sets their own payment rates, and the U.S. government regulates the health care industry on cost and quality. But our checks on costs are nowhere near those of other industrialized nations. For instance, Congress has repeatedly voted down attempts to let Medicare negotiate drug prices (though this changed in 2022, see the Note on the Inflation Reduction Act at the beginning of this book). Whether this relative weakness of regulation is good or bad (and there are strong opinions on both sides), it does contribute to higher costs for patients in the United States.

Low-Value Care

Low-value care is estimated to account for up to $100 billion of annual health care spending.[50] Medical services are defined as low value when they provide little to no clinical benefit yet incur cost. To address this, the American Board of Internal Medicine started the Choosing Wisely Campaign in 2012. Choosing Wisely asks specialty organizations to contribute "top five lists" of services they'd like to see changed, minimized, or stopped altogether; in 2009, they even released a limited list of nonrecommended services in primary care that alone cost an avoidable $6.8 billion.[51]

Medical services may be low value by a variety of mechanisms:

- **Using a Higher Cost Treatment When a Lower Cost Alternative Is Available:** For example, 86% of the avoidable spending listed above comes from using brand names instead of generic forms of statins.[ac]
- **Using a Service That Isn't Medically Necessary:** For example, acute back pain is extremely common and usually resolves on its own; MRIs haven't been shown to be helpful but are still frequently ordered. In 2018, researchers estimated that Medicare alone would save $362 million annually if MRIs weren't ordered for new, acute low back pain.[52] These types of services are typically called overtreatment.[ad]
- **Care in the Wrong Context:** For example, if you've been shot, are having a stroke, or can't breathe, the ED provides an extremely high-value service. That service becomes less valuable, however, if you show up for a cold or chronic knee pain. This is why many public and private insurance plans try to discourage ED use for nonurgent conditions.[ae] The clinic system Community Care of North Carolina offered extra access to their patients, reducing ED visits by 23% and saving Medicaid $161 million in 2006.[53]

Policymakers could set a particular cost–benefit calculation for deciding which services are too low value to cover at all (as England does), but this may fail to account for outliers (those whose bodies and experiences don't fit the average) and patient preference.

High Salaries

When we talk about lowering health care costs, we should remember that a huge chunk of those costs are payments or salaries for health workers. About half of the money spent on health care goes toward salaries, for both professional (ie, physicians and nurses) and nonprofessional (ie, schedulers, patient care technicians) workers[54] (Table 3.3).

Physicians and nurses are paid more in the United States than in most other industrialized nations, and wages for both have increased faster than any other occupation in the past 50 years.[55] Obviously, you can offer many

---

[ac]A class of cholesterol-lowering medications (see Chapter 5).
[ad]See the book *Overtreated* by Shannon Brownlee and New Yorker article "America's Epidemic of Unnecessary Care" by Atul Gawande.
[ae]A tricky issue with its own risks, and which has not been easy to address!

Table 3.3 Salaries for Health Workers

Work type	Median income
Home health aides	$28,060
All U.S. workers	$41,950
Radiology technician	$61,900
Registered nurses	$80,010
Family medicine physicians	$207,380
Orthopedic surgeons	$306,220

Source: Adapted from U.S. Bureau of Labor Statistics. Occupational outlook handbook: Physicians and surgeons. Accessed April 3, 2022. https://www.bls.gov/ooh/healthcare/physicians-and-surgeons.htm

reasons why physicians' and nurses' wages are and should be high (they have incredible responsibility to never make mistakes, they work long hours, their jobs are important to society, they spend many years in training for little or no pay, they have a lot of debt to pay off, and, perhaps most importantly, cutting corners on their care is unlikely to improve quality and outcomes), and you also can argue that some of the other salaries should be higher. But when we discuss lowering health care costs and cutting administrative waste, sometimes what we are really talking about is cutting someone's job and pay. On the flip side, when we discuss quality improvement reforms such as improving nurse staffing ratios, we are also talking about spending more money on salaries for more nurses.

Complex Care Doesn't Come Cheap

We can't expect managing chronic disease for decades, or pulling out all the stops to keep someone with serious illness from dying, to be cheap.

Diabetes, heart disease, cirrhosis, HIV, and emphysema are chronic conditions without a quick cure. Over the decades, they have become less and less deadly, because of incredible but expensive research, pharmaceutical development, and clinical practice improvements, but now they can require expensive treatment for decades (see Figure 3.12).

Let's look at diabetes. Type 2 diabetes is highly genetic but also affected by lifestyle, has a huge variety in severity and outcomes, and can cause severe complications. The prevalence has increased from about 1% of Americans in 1960 to 10.5% in 2020.[56,57] In 1960, the only diabetes medication was insulin, which was advertised at the time at a cost between 84 cents

Average Adult Total Health Spending Based on Diagnosis Status, 2019

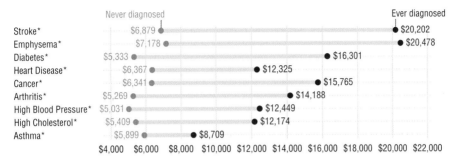

	Never diagnosed	Ever diagnosed
Stroke*	$6,879	$20,202
Emphysema*	$7,178	$20,478
Diabetes*	$5,333	$16,301
Heart Disease*	$6,367	$12,325
Cancer*	$6,341	$15,765
Arthritis*	$5,269	$14,188
High Blood Pressure*	$5,031	$12,449
High Cholesterol*	$5,409	$12,174
Asthma*	$5,899	$8,709

$4,000 $6,000 $8,000 $10,000 $12,000 $14,000 $16,000 $18,000 $20,000 $22,000

Figure 3.12 Note: For diagnoses shown, with the exception of asthma and diabetes, diagnosis status was asked only of respondents age 18 or older. All respondents up to age 85 were asked about their asthma and diabetes diagnosis status. A (*) next to the disease name indicates that there is a statistically significant difference ($P < .05$) between individuals who have ever been diagnosed and never diagnosed with the disease. (Adapted from Ortaliza J, McGough M, Wager E, et al. How do health expenditures vary across the population? *Peterson-KFF Health System Tracker*. Published November 12, 2021. https://www.healthsystemtracker.org/chart-collection/health-expenditures-vary-across-population/)

and $2 per vial[58] (in 2021, that would be $7.78 to $18.53) (see Chapter 5). Today, we have many more types of insulin as well as medication options beyond insulin—but all of these medications have gotten more expensive.[af] Today, people with diabetes have medical spending on average 2.3 times higher than those without,[59] with expenditures of $16,752 annually ($9,601 of which is attributable to diabetes),[60] and in total, diabetes accounts for 3.4% of all health spending.[61] Of course, we can and should spend money to treat diabetes effectively! The point is, the care of chronic disease is expensive, and only getting more so.

Another hot button topic in this category is the cost of end-of-life care. Health spending at the end-of-life greatly outstrips that at any other time; an estimated 13% to 25% of Medicare spending goes to care in the last year of life.[62] Patients, physicians, and families often "pull out all the stops" to treat those near death, even if the tests and procedures have little chance of succeeding. The bioethicist Arthur Caplan states, "What would you do if your mother needed an expensive, painful operation that had only a one in a million chance of saving her? [...] Most Americans would say 'do it.' In this country, we are all about hope."[52]

[af]The rising price of insulin is a whole topic in itself, as discussed further in Chapter 5

Unfortunately, you rarely know ahead of time that it's your last year of life. It's obvious that death is inevitable, and, in hindsight, it seems odd to spend hundreds of thousands of dollars to extend lives by only a few months. Yet, for patients and their families in the moment, impending death may not feel obvious, and a few more months with your loved ones can be precious. Just as inevitable as death is the fact that health care will always be mediated by emotion. Many patients and families seek to pull out all the stops to prolong life. And that's expensive.

Paying for Social Determinants of Health

SDoH are "conditions in the places where people live, learn, work, and play that affect a wide range of health and quality-of life-risks and outcomes."[63] SDoH have become a bigger topic of discussion within health care in the past decade, recognizing that all kinds of external factors in the environment and society affect individual health.

For instance, if you live where there is higher pollution, you'll be more likely to get asthma. If you work manual labor jobs that don't offer ESI or sick leave, you'll have much less access to health care. If you live 100 miles from the closest rheumatologist, your rheumatoid arthritis might get a lot worse. And if you are unhoused, basically every aspect of your health is affected. And those downstream costs might be seen as more inhaler prescriptions, higher rates of late-discovered cancer, more joint surgeries, and higher ED visits and hospital admissions.

And although personal behaviors affect health (such as exercise, diet, and smoking), we can see how social factors influence those behaviors: agricultural and economic policy makes McDonald's cheaper than fresh produce, unsafe neighborhoods discourage people from taking a jog, and the tobacco tax reduces cigarettes sold.

As we showed at the beginning of this chapter, the United States spends far more, as a percentage of GDP, on health than comparable countries, leading some to suggest that the United States pays more for health care *because* we pay less for other social services (like elder care, housing, and disability payments). However, studies have not clearly borne this out, given that countries that spend more on social services also tend to spend more on health care, and given that the United States is about middle of the pack on social spending[64] (Figure 3.13).

Nonetheless, this is in aggregate, and many in public health and medical fields support more funding for better social services as a way to intervene "upstream" to affect "downstream" medical outcomes and, ultimately, costs: for instance, the "Housing First" approach of addressing homelessness.[65]

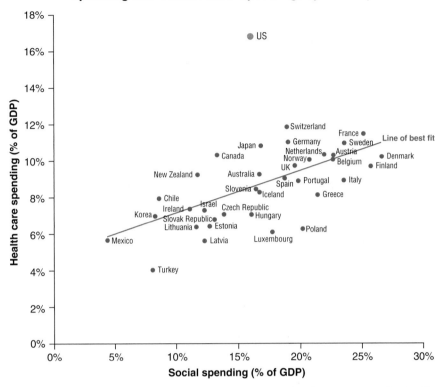

Percent of Gross Domestic Product (GDP) Devoted to Social Spending and Health Care Spending, by Country

Figure 3.13 Adapted from Papanicolas I, Woskie LR, Orlander D, Orav EJ, Jha AK. The relationship between health spending and social spending in high-income countries: how does the US compare? *Health Affairs.* 2019;38(9). https://www.healthaffairs.org/doi/10.1377/hlthaff.2018.05187

Misaligned Incentives

In this book, we've discussed the following groups in the health system:

Patients	Private insurance	Public insurance
Hospitals	Pharmaceutical companies	Public health workers
Pharmacies	Nursing facilities	PBMs
Medical device companies	Policymakers	Health workers (docs, nurses, etc)

All of these groups have their own perspective and interests. One thing they all have in common is they want more money, either by spending less or making more. But in such a complicated system, the actions of one group (in an attempt to maximize their money) can lead to unintended consequences and the ratcheting up of costs. Take a look at some of the issues discussed in this book—such as surprise billing in Chapter 6 or prescription drug rebates in Chapter 5—and think through how the different stakeholders acting in their own interests might drive up overall costs.

"Cost Disease"

As health care costs have risen, costs for other goods such as telecommunications and home appliances have become much cheaper. Economist William Baumol explained this widespread phenomenon by comparing gains in productivity in different sectors of the economy.[66] For example, an American farmer in 2000 produced on average 12 times as much farm output per hour worked as a farmer did in 1950,[67] whereas research shows that, on average, physicians see fewer patients per day now than they did in 1970.[68,69] So, although the farmer's productivity went up by 1,100%, the physician's productivity has decreased—at least in the dimension of number of patients treated in a day.

As productivity in certain industries rises, prices for those products will decrease. As prices decrease in some sectors of the economy, other, less productive sectors become relatively scarcer and thus their prices rise. In general, productivity has increased the most for sectors of the economy that produce tangible goods (like cars, computers, and clothes) and increased the least for sectors of the economy that produce intangible services (like education and health care) (Figure 3.14).

Following the logic of this "cost disease," as Baumol nicknamed the effect, leads to the conclusion that the only way to truly reduce the price of health care would be to increase the productivity of the health care industry. Exactly what that entails—and how to achieve it—is not at all clear. After all, a physician in 2020 is much more effective at keeping her patients healthy, improving their quality of life, and reducing their risk of mortality than her counterparts from 1970. But "efficacy" isn't necessarily "productivity." You might be able to fit a thousand times more transistors on a computer chip than you could in 1970, but talking to someone about their symptoms takes the same amount of time.

Zooming out to even more of a bird's-eye view, we note that despite the massive changes to regulation and delivery of health care in the United States in the past 70 years, despite the fact that health care costs inch up as a proportion of GDP, in fact the *relationship* between GDP and health care spending has held almost exactly constant over time,[ag] as seen in Figure 3.15. Economists like Alex Tabarrok think that how much we pay for health care

---

[ag]For every 1% that GDP per capita rises, health spending per capita rises 2.4%.

Price of Selected Goods and Services 1950-2016

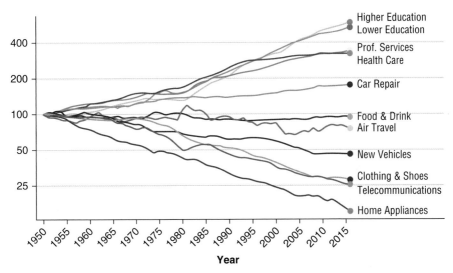

Figure 3.14 Note: Prices normalized to 100 in 1950 Ratio scale. (Adapted from Helland E, Tabarrok A. *Why Are the Prices So D*mn High?* Mercatus Center George Mason University; 2019. https://www.mercatus.org/system/files/helland-tabarrok_why-are-the-prices-so-damn-high_v2.pdf)

is driven by the size of the U.S. economy itself (ie, we pay so much because we can—as we get richer, we spend more on health care), rather than factors internal to the health care system (ie, than any of the other reasons listed in this section).[55]

Health Spending per Capita Versus GDP per capita, 1950-2000

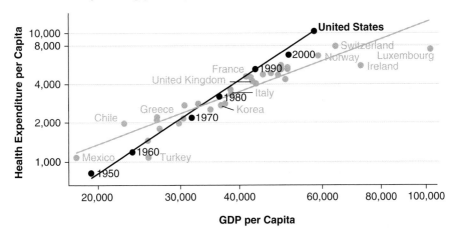

Figure 3.15

Summing It Up

So why do we spend so much on health care? Because our high GDP permits us to pay high prices. Because our government doesn't regulate prices to the extent that other countries do, and because we don't invest as much into improving social drivers of poor health outcomes. Because few individuals have enough or the right information when they need it. Because it's a wild ecosystem with little coordination and with self-interested actors doing their best to get a slice of the pie. Because culture and self-interest affect clinicians' habits and patients' preferences. Because highly trained professionals performing high-stakes jobs don't come cheap. Because high-quality and innovative care doesn't come cheap, either. And because it doesn't really make sense to become more efficient at spending time with someone who needs it.

That's an awful lot of things that need to be addressed by any would-be reformers.

References

1. CMS.gov. NHE Fact Sheet. Published May, 2022. https://www.cms.gov/Research-Statistics-Data-and-Systems/Statistics-Trends-and-Reports/NationalHealthExpendData/NHE-Fact-Sheet

2. The World Bank. All countries and economies. Published May, 2022. https://data.world-bank.org/indicator/NY.GDP.MKTP.CD

3. Health care expenditures per capita by state of residence. *KFF*. State Health Facts. Published April, 2022. https://www.kff.org/other/state-indicator/health-spending-per-capita/?current Timeframe=0&sortModel=%7B%22colId%22:%22Location%22,%22sort%22:%22asc %22%7D

4. BEA. Interactive data. Interactive access to industry economic accounts data. Published June, 2022. https://apps.bea.gov/iTable/iTable.cfm?reqid=150&step=2&isuri= 1&categories=gdpxind

5. Mitchell EM. Statistical Brief #533: concentration of healthcare expenditures and selected characteristics of high spenders, U.S. civilian noninstitutionalized population, 2018. Agency for Healthcare Research and Quality. Published January 2021. https://meps.ahrq.gov/data_files/publications/st533/stat533.shtml

6. Cohn J. Cause for concern: health-care costs are rising—and the experts aren't sure why. Accessed July 8, 2014. www.newrepublic.com/article/117452/rising-health-care-costs-what-it-means-economy-obamacare

7. Holahan J, Blumberg LJ, Clemans-Cope L, et al. The evidence on recent health care spending growth and the impact of the affordable care act. *Robert Wood Johnson Foundation*. Published May, 2017. http://www.urban.org/sites/default/files/publication/90471/2001288-the_evidence_on_recent_health_care_spending_growth_and_the_impact_of_the_affordable_care_act.pdf

8. Jaffe S. No more secrets: Congress bans pharmacist 'Gag Orders' on drug prices. *KHN*. Published October 10, 2018. https://khn.org/news/no-more-secrets-congress-bans-pharmacist-gag-orders-on-drug-prices/

9. Singer P. Why we must ration health care. *New York Times*. Published July 15, 2009. https://www.nytimes.com/2009/07/19/magazine/19healthcare-t.html

10. Porter ME, Teisberg EO. *Redefining Health Care: Creating Value-Based Competition on Results*. Harvard Business School Press; 2006.

11. Roy A. Why the American Medical Association had 72 million reasons to shrink doctors' pay. *Forbes*. Published November 28, 2011. https://www.forbes.com/sites/theapothecary/2011/11/28/why-the-american-medical-association-had-72-million-reasons-to-help-shrink-doctors-pay/?sh=380bedab60d9

12. National average payment table update. *Optum*. July, 2022. https://www.optumcoding.com/upload/docs/2021%20DRG_National%20Average%20Payment%20Table_Update.pdf

13. Stanford hospital accused of alleged $468 million dollar healthcare billing fraud: DOJ filed its statement of interest in federal court. *AP News*. Published June 19, 2020. https://apnews.com/press-release/prcom/business-72b885fd050ba0f7512fc942457b3647

14. Frakt A. Hospitals are wrong for shifting costs to private insurers. The Upshot. *The New York Times*. Published March 23, 2015. https://www.nytimes.com/2015/03/24/upshot/why-hospitals-are-wrong-about-shifting-costs-to-private-insurers.html?rref=upshot&abt=0002&abg=1

15. Roy A. @Avik. Twitter Web Client. May 10, 2019. https://twitter.com/Avik/status/1126953046628601856?s=20

16. Kliff S, Katz J. Hospitals and insurers didn't want you to see these prices. Here's why. The Upshot. *The New York Times*. Published August 22, 2021. https://www.nytimes.com/interactive/2021/08/22/upshot/hospital-prices.html?campaign_id=9&emc=edit_nn_20210823&instance_id=38591&nl=the-morning&regi_id=69542217&segment_id=66986&te=1&user_id=f32bb8e73abca4414430586c0307cd4c

17. Reinhardt UE. *Priced Out*. 1st ed. Princeton University Press; 2019.

18. *APM Measurement: Progress of Alternative Payment Models*. 2021. HCPlan. http://hcp-lan.org/workproducts/APM-Methodology-2020-2021.pdf

19. Managed care: what went wrong? Can it be fixed? *Stanford Business*. Published November 01, 1999. https://www.gsb.stanford.edu/insights/managed-care-what-went-wrong-can-it-be-fixed

20. Biniek JF, Cubanski J, Neuman T. Higher and faster growing spending per Medicare advantage enrollee adds to Medicare's solvency and affordability challenges. *KFF*. Published August 17, 2021. https://www.kff.org/medicare/issue-brief/higher-and-faster-growing-spending-per-medicare-advantage-enrollee-adds-to-medicares-solvency-and-affordability-challenges/

21. Muhlestein D, Bleser WK, Saunders RS, McClellan MB. All-payer spread of ACOs and value-based payment models in 2021: the crossroads and future of value-based care. *Health Affairs*. Published June 17, 2021. https://www.healthaffairs.org/do/10.1377/hblog20210609.824799/full/

22. The Dartmouth Institute for Health Policy & Clinical Practice. National survey of accountable care organizations. Published July, 2022. https://tdi.dartmouth.edu/research/our-research/accountable-care-organizations/national-survey-acos

23. NAACOS. National Association of ACOs. https://www.naacos.com/

24. CMS.gov. Affordable Care Act's shared savings program continues to improve quality of care while saving Medicare money during the COVID-19 pandemic. Published August 25,

2021. https://www.cms.gov/newsroom/press-releases/affordable-care-acts-shared-savings-program-continues-improve-quality-care-while-saving-medicare

25. McWilliams JM, Landon BE, Rathi VK, Chernew ME. Getting more savings from ACOs—can the pace be pushed? *N Engl J Med.* 2019;380(23):2190-2192. doi:10.1056/NEJMp1900537. https://www.ncbi.nlm.nih.gov/pmc/articles/PMC6624070/

26. Glass D, McClendon S, Stensland J. Long-term issues confronting Medicare Accountable Care Organizations (ACOs). *Medpac.* Published April 6, 2018. https://www.medpac.gov/wp-content/uploads/import_data/scrape_files/docs/default-source/default-document-library/aco_april-2018.pdf

27. Medpac. Chapter 12: The Medicare Advantage program: status report. Published March, 2021. https://www.medpac.gov/wp-content/uploads/2021/10/mar21_medpac_report_ch12_sec.pdf

28. The United States Department of Justice. Medicare advantage provider to pay $270 million to settle false claims act liabilities. Published October 1, 2018. https://www.justice.gov/opa/pr/medicare-advantage-provider-pay-270-million-settle-false-claims-act-liabilities

29. Kaiser permanents defrauded Medicare of $1 billion, DOJ alleges. *Bloomberg Law.* Published October 26, 2021. https://news.bloomberglaw.com/health-law-and-business/kaiser-permanente-defrauded-medicare-of-1-billion-doj-alleges

30. Jacobson G, Fehr R, Cox C, Neuman T. Financial performance of Medicare advantage, individual, and group health insurance markets. *KFF.* Published August 5, 2019. https://www.kff.org/report-section/financial-performance-of-medicare-advantage-individual-and-group-health-insurance-markets-issue-brief/

31. Medpac. Report to the Congress. Medicare and the health care delivery system. Published June, 2021. https://www.medpac.gov/wp-content/uploads/import_data/scrape_files/docs/default-source/reports/jun21_medpac_report_to_congress_sec.pdf

32. Schwartz AL, Zlaoui K, Foreman RP, Brennan TA, Newhouse JP. Health care utilization and spending in Medicare advantage vs traditional Medicare: a difference-in-differences analysis. *JAMA Health Forum.* 2021;2(12):e214001. doi:10.1001/jamahealthforum.2021.4001. https://jamanetwork.com/journals/jama-health-forum/fullarticle/2787081

33. Medpac. Skilled nursing facility services payment system. Revised November, 2021. https://www.medpac.gov/wp-content/uploads/2021/11/medpac_payment_basics_21_snf_final_sec.pdf

34. Murray C, Tourtellotte A, Lipson D, Wysocki A. *Medicaid Long Term Services and Supports Annual Expenditures Report: Federal Fiscal Years 2017 and 2018.* Mathematica; 2021.

35. Consolidation in California's health care market 2010-2016: impact on prices and ACA premiums. Nicholas C. Petris Center on Health Care Markets and Consumer Welfare. School of Public Health. University of California, Berkeley. Published March 26, 2018. http://petris.org/wp-content/uploads/2018/03/CA-Consolidation-Full-Report_03.26.18.pdf

36. Zhu JM, Polsky D. Private equity and physician medical practices—navigating a changing ecosystem. *N Engl J Med.* 2021;384:981-983. doi:10.1056/NEJMp2032115

37. Kane CK. Policy research perspectives. Updated data on physician practice arrangements: for the first time, fewer physicians are owners than employees. *American Medical Association.* 2019. https://www.ama-assn.org/system/files/2019-07/prp-fewer-owners-benchmark-survey-2018.pdf

38. Fulton, Brent, D. Health Care Market Concentration Trends in the United States: Evidence and Policy Responses. *Health Affairs.* September 2017. https://www.healthaffairs.org/doi/10.1377/hlthaff.2017.0556

39. Gold J. Surprise settlement in Sutter health antitrust case. *California Healthline.* Published October 16, 2019. https://californiahealthline.org/news/surprise-settlement-in-sutter-health-antitrust-case/

40. Gaynor M, Town R. The synthesis project. *Robert Wood Johnson Foundation.* Published June, 2012. https://citeseerx.ist.psu.edu/viewdoc/download?doi=10.1.1.592.7610&rep=rep1&type=pdf

41. Paavola A. Sutter Health's $575M antitrust settlement is final: 4 things to know. *Becker's Hospital Review.* Updated August 31, 2021. https://www.beckershospitalreview.com/legal-regulatory-issues/sutter-health-s-575m-antitrust-settlement-is-final-4-things-to-know.html

42. Medpac. June, 2022 report to the Congress: Medicare and the health care delivery system. Published June 15, 2022. https://www.medpac.gov/document/june-2022-report-to-the-congress-medicare-and-the-health-care-delivery-system/

43. Appelbaum E, Batt R. Private equity buyouts in healthcare: who wins, who loses? Institute for New Economic Thinking Working Paper Series No. 118. SSRN. doi:10.36687/inetwp118. Published March 15, 2020. https://papers.ssrn.com/sol3/papers.cfm?abstract_id=3593887

44. Dark Daily. UnitedHealth Group soon to be largest employer of doctors in the US; clinical laboratory outreach more critical than ever before. Published June 29, 2018. https://www.darkdaily.com/2018/06/29/unitedhealth-group-soon-to-be-largest-employer-of-doctors-in-the-us-clinical-laboratory-outreach-more-critical-than-ever-before-629/#:~:text=Pending%20the%20successful%20completion%20of,numbers%20reported%20by%20leading%20sources

45. NAIC. Pharmacy Benefit Managers. Updated April 11, 2022. https://content.naic.org/cipr_topics/topic_pharmacy_benefit_managers.htm; Cassity A. NAIC Pharmacy Benefit Manager Regulatory Issues Subgroup Pharmacist Industry Perspective. National Community Pharmacists Association (NCPA). August, 2019.

46. Visante. Pharmacy Benefit Managers (PBMs): generating savings for plan sponsors and consumers. *PCMA.* Published February 2020. https://www.pcmanet.org/wp-content/uploads/2020/02/Pharmacy-Benefit-Managers-Generating-Savings-for-Plan-Sponsors-and-Consumers-2020-1.pdf

47. The Commonwealth Fund. Pharmacy benefit managers and their role in drug spending. Published April 22, 2019. https://www.commonwealthfund.org/publications/explainer/2019/apr/pharmacy-benefit-managers-and-their-role-drug-spending

48. Anderson G, Hussey P, Petrosyan V. It's still the prices, stupid: why the US spends so much on health care, and a tribute to Uwe Reinhardt. *Health Affairs.* 2019;38(1):87-95. doi:10.1377/hlthaff.2018.05144. ©2019 Project HOPE—The People-to-People Health Foundation, Inc. https://www.healthaffairs.org/doi/pdf/10.1377/hlthaff.2018.05144

49. Although the Hospital readmission reduction program did aim to improve this. See the Case Study on Hospital Readmissions at the end of this book.

50. Shrank WH, Rogstad TL, Parekh N. Waste in the US health care system: estimated costs and potential for savings. *JAMA.* 2019;322(15):1501-1509. doi:10.1001/jama.2019.13978

51. Kale MS, Bishop TF, Federman AD, Keyhani S. "Top 5" lists top $5 billion. *Arch Intern Med.* 2011;171(20):1858-1859. doi:10.1001/archinternmed.2011.501

52. Garber A, Azad TD, Dixit A, et al. Medicare savings from conservative management of low back pain. *Am J Manag Care.* 2018;24(10):e332-e337. https://www.ajmc.com/view/medicare-savings-from-conservative-management-of-low-back-pain

53. Steiner BD, Denham AC, Ashkin E, Newton WP, Wroth T, Dobson LA Jr. Community care of North Carolina: improving care through community health networks. *Ann Fam Med.* 2008;6(4):361-367. doi:10.1370/afm.866. https://www.annfammed.org/content/6/4/361.long

54. Glied SA, Ma S, Pearlstein I. Understanding pay differentials among health professionals, nonprofessionals, and their counterparts in other sectors. *Health Affairs*. Published June, 2015. https://www.healthaffairs.org/doi/10.1377/hlthaff.2014.1367

55. Helland E, Tabarrok A. *Why Are the Prices So D*mn High?* Mercatus Center George Mason University; 2019. https://www.mercatus.org/system/files/helland-tabarrok_why-are-the-prices-so-damn-high_v2.pdf

56. Long-term trends in diabetes. Published April, 2017. https://www.cdc.gov/diabetes/statistics/slides/long_term_trends.pdf

57. Centers for Disease Control and Prevention. National diabetes statistics report. Estimates of diabetes and its burden in the United States. Accessed July, 2022. https://www.cdc.gov/diabetes/data/statistics-report/index.html?CDC_AA_refVal=https%3A%2F%2Fwww.cdc.gov%2Fdiabetes%2Fdata%2Fstatistics%2Fstatistics-report.html

58. Johnson C. Why treating diabetes keeps getting more expensive. *The Washington Post*. Published October 31, 2016. https://www.washingtonpost.com/news/wonk/wp/2016/10/31/why-insulin-prices-have-kept-rising-for-95-years/

59. Petersen MP. Economic costs of diabetes in the U.S. in 2017. *Diabetes Care*. 2018; 41(5):917-928. doi:10.2337/dci18-0007

60. American Diabetes Association. The cost of diabetes. 2022. https://www.diabetes.org/resources/statistics/cost-diabetes

61. Kamal R, Kurani N, Ramirez M, Gonzales S. How have diabetes costs and outcomes changed over time in the U.S.? *Peterson-KFF Health System Tracker*. Published November 15, 2019. https://www.healthsystemtracker.org/chart-collection/diabetes-care-u-s-changed-time/#item-usdiabetes_diabetes-medications-were-second-among-conditions-for-drug-spending-in-2018

62. Duncan I, Ahmed T, Dove H, Maxwell TL. Medicare cost at end of life. *Am J Hosp Palliat Care*. 2019;36(8):705-710. doi:10.1177/1049909119836204

63. Centers for Disease Control and Prevention. Social determinants of health: know what affects health. Accessed July, 2022. https://www.cdc.gov/socialdeterminants/index.htm

64. Papanicolas I, Woskie LR, Orlander D, Orav EJ, Jha AK. The relationship between health spending and social spending in high-income countries: how does the US compare? *Health Affairs*. 2019;38(9). https://doi.org/10.1377/hlthaff.2018.05187

65. Kertesz SG, Baggett TP, O'Connell JJ, et al. Permanent Supportive housing for homeless people—reframing the debate. *N Engl J Med*. 2016;375:2115-2117. doi:10.1056/NEJMp1608326

66. Baumol WJ, de Ferranti D, Malach M, et al. *The Cost Disease: Why Computers Get Cheaper and Health Care Doesn't*. Illustrated edition. Yale University Press; 2013. https://www.amazon.com/Cost-Disease-Computers-Cheaper-Health/dp/0300198159

67. Fuglie KO, MacDonald JM, Ball E. Productivity growth in U.S. agriculture. Economic Brief Number 9. United States Department of Agriculture. Published September, 2007. https://www.ers.usda.gov/webdocs/publications/42924/11854_eb9_1_.pdf

68. *2018 Survey of America's Physicians: Practice Patterns & Perspectives*. The Physicians Foundation. Published September, 2018. https://physiciansfoundation.org/wp-content/uploads/2018/09/physicians-survey-results-final-2018.pdf

69. Mechanic D. The organization of medical practice and practice orientations among physicians in prepaid and nonprepaid primary care settings. *Med Care*. 1975;13(3):189-204. doi:10.1097/00005650-197503000-00001

4

Quality and Technology

Questions as you read through the chapter:

1. How do you define "quality"? What makes medical care high quality to you?
2. What can technology make better in medicine? What can it make worse?
3. The rise of both quality improvement and health technology has produced a lot of data, in many different realms. Who should own this data? Who should be responsible for data reporting? For organizing data?
4. What makes a good incentive? How should a system set incentives?
5. A physician or nurse juggles a lot of different tasks at any given moment. What tasks should be done by a human, and what by a machine? What role does human psychology play in complicated systems like health care?

Why are quality and technology combined in one chapter? At first glance, they may not seem like connected topics. Yet both are relatively new fields that exploded within the past 25 years to shape the way care is delivered in the 2020s. In practice, they feed into each other as interdependent methods trying to make medical care better. They are also aspirational: our technological capabilities and our knowledge of what the best care looks like often far outpace the current capabilities of the delivery and reimbursement system.

Quality and Safety

Medical care can be of variable quality and can even do harm. Paying attention to the quality of medical services is not a new concept. In the 19th century, Florence Nightingale began asking medical staff to wash their hands to reduce infections, and in the early 20th century, the American College of

Surgeons began auditing their members' quality. But the concept of medical quality as a field of study *is* relatively new. Its birth is often dated to 1999, when the Institute of Medicine (IOM) published a report called *To Err Is Human: Building a Safer Health System.*[1] This famous report stated that "errors are common, they are costly, systems-related problems cause errors, errors can be prevented, and safety can be improved."[2] The report also made the shocking claim that medical errors lead to 46,000 to 98,000[a] deaths every year, making medical errors a major cause of mortality in America.

Patient safety and quality is now a huge field, with entire hospital divisions, payment and bonus metrics, and many organizations dedicated to it. This field borrowed from similar tactics in other industries—like aviation—to develop systematic approaches to defining errors (or problems) and measuring improvement. For the decade or so after *To Err Is Human*, efforts focused on reducing obvious areas in which medical care caused harm, such as hospital-acquired infections and medication errors, and on leveraging technology such as electronic health records (EHRs) to track quality. We've had some huge improvements, though much remains to improve (including, perhaps, the methods of quality improvement).[2] More recently, quality improvement efforts have expanded beyond "doing less harm" to "doing more good," in areas such as preventive care and equity.

Let's review some definitions, standard approaches, and specific areas of focus in quality improvement.

Definitions

Defining quality is notoriously difficult. Let's start with the basics and the big picture. Here, we'll define safety, quality, value, and systems improvement. These terms overlap and are often used interchangeably, but they are slightly different.

Safety is basically the first part of the Hippocratic Oath: First, do no harm. Or, as the Agency for Healthcare Research and Quality (AHRQ) puts it, "freedom from accidental or preventable injuries produced by medical care."[3] Patient safety focuses on reducing errors, which can range from extremely important to not-so-important (Table 4.1).

In contrast to safety, *quality* isn't just freedom from error: it's about doing things well, "doing the right thing at the right time in the right way for the right person and having the best results possible."[5] The IOM defines the six specific aims of high-quality care as safe, effective, patient-centered, timely, efficient, and equitable.[4] Sounds great! But in order to track and measure quality

---

[a]If that strikes you as a big range, don't worry—you're not the first to notice. These figures from the IOM have been disputed and are controversial.

Table 4.1 Types of Medical Errors

Type	Definition[a]	Example
Sentinel events (and never events)	Serious adverse events involving death or serious physiologic or psychological injury, or the risk thereof	Amputating the wrong leg
Adverse event (preventable)	Harm from medical care rather than an underlying disease; occurred because of error or failure to adhere to the accepted standard of care	Pressure ulcer after not turning the patient frequently enough
Adverse event (nonpreventable)	Harm occurred despite care adhering to the accepted standard of care (ie, no negligence)	Pressure ulcer despite maximal preventive measures
Near miss	An unsafe situation that is indistinguishable from a preventable adverse event except for the outcome	Accidentally giving aspirin to a patient with a recent head bleed, but luckily no further bleeding occurred
Error	A general umbrella term referring to any act of doing something wrong—or failing to add a preventive step—that exposes a patient to potential or actual harm	Prescribing two medications with a bad potential drug interaction

AHRQ, Agency for Healthcare Research and Quality.
[a]All definitions taken from AHRQ's Patient Safety Network. https://psnet.ahrq.gov/

improvement, you have to get much more precise about these adjectives, which are highly context dependent. Let's say you want to improve the mammogram screening rate: you need to specifically define who warrants mammogram screening, the frequency with which you think they should get mammograms, and who is overdue for a mammogram. When you take action—say, sending automated reminder letters—you need to check whether this actually did improve the rate, and if it did so for all people or only worked for some.[b]

Sometimes quality is tracked internally but frequently it is defined and tracked externally, by the state and by payers—especially Medicare. These external measures very frequently focus on standards of care, such as cancer screenings, chronic disease management, and preventable errors. We'll talk more about external measures later.

---

[b]Then working with the research system to evaluate whether more cases of breast cancer were identified, and if this actually improved mortality.

Another term that sometimes gets conflated with quality is *value*. Whereas safety and quality is a system of measurement and improvement of outcomes, value is maximizing those outcomes at lower or similar cost. Another way of putting this is the "Triple Aim," popularized by the Institute for Healthcare Improvement, recognizing that health care should aim to "improve the patient experience of care, improve the health of populations, and reduce the per capita cost of care."[c,5] As such, value is a major concept for alternative payment models (APMs), which are sometimes also called "value-based care" (see Chapter 3).

Delivering medical care is complicated, and many, many elements of care contribute to safety, quality, and value. Most often, you can't improve quality, safety, and value through the actions of just one person. Rather, you need *systems improvement*.

Any lecture on health care quality will show some version of this "Swiss cheese" graphic (Figure 4.1), which demonstrates that, typically, more than one thing has to go wrong for an error to occur, and that adverse events can occur despite multiple barriers. Most errors aren't because of just one person messing up but, rather, occur because of deficiencies within the incredibly complex health care delivery system. Think of a large hospital—a fast-paced, stressful environment with thousands of employees and a dizzying array of computer systems and medical devices. It's easy to imagine how a small miscommunication or oversight might combine with another small mistake, leading to an unintended event.

Thus, efforts to stem medical errors don't simply target errors by individuals but often focus on improving health care system design and on enhancing

Swiss Cheese Model of Medical Errors

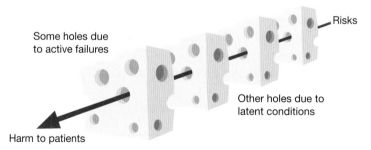

Figure 4.1 Adapted from Reason JT, Carthey J, de Leval MR. Diagnosing "vulnerable system syndrome": an essential prerequisite to effective risk management. *Qual Health Care*. 2001;10(suppl 2):ii21-ii25. doi:10.1136/qhc.0100021

---

[c]Sometimes also called the Quadruple Aim, including improved clinician experience, as well.

the transfer of information between providers. Eliminating human error is impossible; instead, the key should be creating a safe system where human errors are anticipated and prevented. *To Err Is Human* suggests that "mistakes can best be prevented by designing the health system at all levels to make it safer—to make it harder for people to do something wrong and easier for them to do it right."[1]

Measurement and Action

It's concerning when you hear that 50,000+ people might be dying a year from medical errors, or that American life expectancy stalled out and has gotten worse than peer nations since 2014,[6] or that Americans receive only about 55% of all recommended care.[7] But you can't just say, "hey, let's make people live longer" and expect to be successful. Instead, quality improvement work focuses narrowly on a systematic approach to specific, definable, and actionable problems. Let's learn a little about the nature of this work.

Big picture: Donabedian triad

The "Donabedian triad" is a commonly used framework for how to measure quality. The triad is structure, process, and outcomes.

Let's start first with *outcomes* (ie, what happened to the patient after care was delivered?). Of course, this is what we care about the most. However, outcomes can take a long time to come to fruition, meaning that we might wait years or even decades to understand our successes or failures. An example of this might be, what percentage of patients are still alive a year after heart surgery?

We can monitor *process* (ie, what care was delivered and how?) on a shortened time scale, making it easier to focus on than outcomes. For instance, how many of those heart surgery patients received appropriate antibiotics before surgery?

Finally, we can evaluate *structure* (ie, what is the organization like that delivered the care?), which includes elements such as staffing, finances, and resourcing. To continue our example of heart surgery patients, what is the nurse staffing ratio for postoperative patients?

Measuring safety

Errors occur in every setting, but here let's look at the hospital, using an example in which a patient's central line (ie, a type of intravenous catheter inserted into a large vein and going close to the patient's heart) was left in too long. Sometimes when this happens, a patient gets a bloodstream infection. Central line–associated bloodstream infections (CLABSIs) are a big deal and have been a major focus of quality improvement work.

If we are tracking quality of care in the hospital, first, how do we know an error occurred? Traditionally, through things like incident reports, in which someone who notices the error reports it to the system. A nurse might then report either a concern about a central line placement or infection. However, generally speaking, far fewer errors get reported than occur. If you know what you're looking for, errors can also be identified through trigger tools, reviews of complications, and EHR data. Bedside nurses have long been the eyes and ears of the quality system, but technology increasingly helps out.

Second, do we then report the error anywhere? Some errors are only reported within the health system or the hospital tracking them. Others are reported and monitored at the state or even national level. CLABSI rates are tracked by the Centers for Disease Control and Prevention (CDC) nationally, both in terms of specific types of errors (like not following guidelines in insertion) as well as overall rates.

Third, how do we know what caused the error? For an error like leaving in a central line for too long, probably more than one thing contributed. To assess for every contributing factor, quality improvement teams use tools (or investigative guides) like a fishbone—or Ishikawa—diagram (Figure 4.2[8]),

Example of an Ishikawa or "Fishbone" Diagram

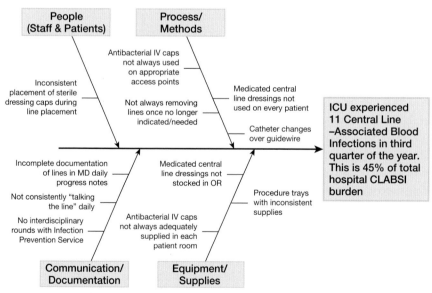

Figure 4.2 CLABSI, central line–associated bloodstream infection; ICU, intensive care unit; IV, intravenous; OR, operating room. (Adapted from Russell TA, Fritschel E, Do J, et al. Minimizing central line–associated bloodstream infections in a high-acuity liver transplant intensive care unit. *Am J Infect Control.* 2019;47(3):305-312. doi:10.1016/j.ajic.2018.08.006)

root cause analysis, or asking the Five Whys. Increasingly, health care also uses systematic improvement models borrowed from business, such as Lean and Six Sigma. The older and more traditional method in health care is the Morbidity and Mortality (M&M) conference, in which physicians review a bad outcome—usually a death—and the elements that led to it.

Fourth, what do we do about these errors? Once the health system has identified errors—or factors that lead to bad outcomes—then it should help prevent them! Mostly, prevention or improvement efforts focus on process and structure, as mentioned in the Donabedian triad. The method of prevention depends a lot on what is being prevented and where, but one example is checklists for processes such as inserting and maintaining central lines. In the case of CLABSI, these checklist efforts have helped, and CLABSI rates have decreased significantly: from ~43,000 in 2001[9] to ~21,000 in 2020.[10]

Finally, how do we improve the overall system that leads to errors? There is not a simple fix for errors within a large and complex system. As Lucien Leape says, "the key is recognizing that changing practice is not a technical problem that can be solved by ticking off boxes on a checklist but a social problem of human behavior and interaction."[11] To develop a culture of safety, many health care systems have created positions such as chief quality officer and taken steps to become a "learning health system."[12]

Connection with technology

All of this quality improvement work rests on a foundation of technology. We do not have to flip through thick paper charts to manually collect information, nor rely on clinicians to recognize problems. Rather, EHRs make it possible to extract data, track it, and even to alert clinical teams and prevent errors.

EHRs are very good at some elements of quality measurement and action. For instance, they are great at tracking what's called "discrete" data—like lab values, vital signs, International Classification of Diseases (ICD)-10 diagnoses, how many days a central line was left in, etc. However, much discrete data still need manual input by clinicians and staff (like the date of central line insertion, or giving some exam findings in a questionnaire format rather than free text), which can be a burden.

Plus, not all problems are easily captured in data. Let's say that you are trying to improve diabetes care in your clinic. Your clinic has a lot of patients with blood sugar that is both too high and, at times, too low. In creating your Ishikawa diagram, you realize that a major cause of this is that many patients don't understand how to use their diabetes medications or check their blood sugar at home. You decide to hire a health educator who can work with all patients with diabetes to truly understand their disease and its management. This process measure—patient understanding—is much harder to measure than others, like lab values or how many patients see a health educator. Even if you tried to turn it into checking a box, such as "patient demonstrates understanding," is tracking that statement really going to be an accurate reflection of the messy process of educating?

Sometimes we track what we can, even if it's not the primary goal. In this way, the EHR revolutionizes quality measurement while also limiting the focus of quality improvement to that which is easily measurable.

Quality metrics

Earlier, we mentioned that CLABSI rates get reported to the federal government. In fact, many error rates and quality measures get reported externally, either to the government or to nongovernmental organizations. The most prominent organization defining quality metrics is the National Committee for Quality Assurance, which tracks and compares quality and safety levels between hospitals in their Healthcare Effectiveness Data and Information Set.[d]

There has been an explosion of quality measures in the past 10 to 20 years, particularly with the rise of value-based payment (see Section "APMs and Value-Based Payment" in Chapter 3), as payers seek to include quality measures performance as an element of reimbursement. Between 2008 and 2018, the Centers for Medicare & Medicaid Services (CMS) invested $1.3 billion into the development and use of quality measures, and by the end of that period *788* measures were used in CMS programs.[13] These have since been pared down, but providers still must track and report dozens of measures.

The explosion in metrics tied to reimbursement and quality ratings has led some to question whether they actually impact the overall quality of care. Namely, the focus on tracking may detract from a focus on the patients themselves. Research and surveys in the mid-2010s found that outpatient clinics were spending 15 hours per physician per week on quality reporting,[14] and that health systems hired on average 17 information technology workers for every 100 physicians.[15]

Patient voices do not get lost in all of this. Patient experience is an important category of quality measures. Patients are sent long surveys about their experience after visits and hospitalizations, and the averages are used to compare providers. As an example, 7 out of 33 measures for Medicare accountable care organizations are focused on patient experience.[16]

---

[d]These measures are used frequently by CMS and by APMs in value-based care, but there are many other options for quality measures, as well.

Some Major Areas of Focus in Quality

Learning about quality improvement as a process can feel very abstract without the particular context of a problem. So let's turn to some major areas of quality improvement work. In this section, we review a few major topics in health care quality, while limiting ourselves to two paragraphs each. Think of this as a peek into the kinds of things a chief quality officer might have on their mind.

Medication Errors

Medications save and improve lives, but they also cause harm. This can be due to the inherent risks of the drug itself, as well as errors with prescribing, dispensing, and administering medications. Every year, over 10% of patients in the hospital, and over 7 million patients overall, are affected by a medication error.[17] Adverse drug events (ADEs) prompt 3.5 million clinician office visits, 1 million emergency department (ED) visits, and 125,000 hospital admissions each year.[18] Then, in the hospital itself, nearly 5% of patients experience an ADE.[19] Disturbingly, the totality of medication errors—both in the hospital and out—is estimated to cause 7,000 deaths a year.[20]

Technology has helped to improve quality and reduce ADEs, not only by getting rid of messy doctors' handwriting on prescription pads (yes, a real driver of error in the past!) but also by providing prescribing alerts (such as for allergies and drug interactions) in the EHR, requiring barcode scanning in pharmacies and by nurses, and forcing medication "reconciliation" when a patient enters, transfers between, or leaves the hospital. Medication reconciliation or "med rec," which aims to find and resolve discrepancies between patients' medication lists (at home vs in the hospital, between one health system and another, etc), is hugely important. Research has uncovered evidence of discrepancies in medication lists in about one-half of hospital admissions and in 40% of hospital discharges.[21] Although many organizations and federal quality metrics incentivize medication reconciliation, it remains a difficult and labor-intensive process, and there is no single accepted way to accomplish it.

Health Care–Associated Infections

Health care–associated infections (HAIs), also called nosocomial infections, are those that arise because of the presence of the patient in a health care facility, or to the care received there. HAIs are more likely to happen in people who are severely ill, who have invasive procedures (including bladder catheters and intravenous lines), and when clinicians and staff overuse antibiotics or do not follow standard-of-care practices. The CDC tracks CLABSIs, catheter-associated urinary tract infections, surgical site infections, certain resistant bloodstream infections, ventilator-associated enterococcus, and *Clostridium difficile* diarrhea. Dr Peter Pronovost revolutionized the approach to such infections, by using checklists. Checklists help ensure clinicians and staff don't forget all the little things they are supposed to do, reducing cognitive burden and simplifying complex tasks. The checklist approach had a dramatic effect on HAIs.[22]

Although there was great progress in reducing the rates of these infections in the decade from the mid-2000s to the mid-2010s, still, on any given day in a hospital, 1 out of every 31 patients has an HAI.[23] Total societal costs from HAIs number around $40 billion annually.[e] In an effort to improve quality and lower costs, Medicare has not reimbursed hospitals for any care related to six categories of HAIs, such as surgical site infections after bariatric surgeries, since 2008.[24] Another initiative seeks to make HAIs transparent: Medicare publicly reports rates of some HAIs,[f] and many states require hospitals to report their HAI rates. In addition to a hospital's desire to take better care of their patients, both payment refusal and transparency are incentives to prevent HAIs.

Transitions in Care

Hospitalized patients are sick and complex, and there's a lot to know about them. In the hospital, health care workers (nurses, doctors, pharmacists, etc) can't work 100% of the time, much to the chagrin of hospital chief financial officers (CFOs), so there must be reliable communication about active medical problems, treatments, and issues to anticipate. Nurses do handoffs at the beginning and end of every shift. For doctors, particularly residents, it is a little more complicated, including "cross coverage," in which one intern might oversee 50 or more patients overnight. One study found that any given patient experienced 15 handoffs between residents during a 5-day hospitalization, and a resident physician participated in 300 handoffs during a month-long rotation.[25] Different standardized methods have been developed—such as "SBAR" or "IPASS"[26]—but there is no single standard for clinician or nurse handoffs. Additionally, there is a balance between the risks of fatigue (ie, shift length and duty hours) versus the risks of errors because of frequent handoffs. For example, if you took a turn for the worse overnight in the hospital, would you rather be seen by a physician who knows your medical history but has been awake for 24 hours, or by a physician who is well-rested but you've never met?

---

[e]The CDC reports $28.4 billion in direct medical costs and $12.4 billion in indirect costs to society, such as lost wages. https://www.cdc.gov/policy/polaris/healthtopics/hai/index.html.
[f]You can check them out for yourself at HospitalCompare.hhs.gov.

Transitions also refer to leaving the hospital. This is a vulnerable time, particularly because so many patients are discharged with new diagnoses and medicines, test results pending, part of their diagnostic workup to be completed as an outpatient, and with family members who are expected to provide care without proper—or any—training. Studies have shown that nearly 20% of patients experience an adverse event within 3 weeks of discharge—the majority of which could have been prevented.[27] As such, many health systems have added programs to reduce the risk of transitions home through discharge education, scheduling follow-up visits before the patient leaves the hospital, remote monitoring, home visits, and good old-fashioned telephone calls[28] (see the Case Study on Hospital Readmissions at the end of this book).

Preventive Care

Preventive care includes cancer screenings, immunizations, and counseling on things like alcohol use and exercise. By the early 2000s, reports indicated that, on average, Americans received just over half of recommended preventive care services,[7] and rates have not improved much since then.[29] The rate of adults receiving *all* recommended prevention is quite low—generally 10% or less.[30] Most of these rates have worsened during the pandemic; for instance, breast and cervical cancer screening rates dropped ~85% from 2019 to 2020,[31] and some fear that immunization rates will suffer long term.

This is an area in which social determinants of health loom large, and we see big disparities; for instance, Whites are 12% more likely to get colorectal cancer screening than are Native Americans, and those with a graduate degree are 23% more likely to do so than those without a high school diploma.[32] What reasons contribute to low rates of recommended services, and whose responsibility is it to improve them? With the idea that cost was keeping many people from preventive care, the Affordable Care Act mandated full coverage for a broad array of preventive care services (ie, screening colonoscopies, Pap smears), usually without a copay or deductible. More recently, value-based payment models have shifted responsibility for completing preventive services from individual patients onto health systems (and particularly primary care clinicians) through APMs (see Chapters 1 and 2).

Chronic Disease Management: Spotlight on Hypertension

Hypertension is common—about 50% of adults have it[33]—and can be serious, leading to complications like kidney disease, strokes, and heart failure. High-quality care "controls" blood pressure (BP) below a standard threshold in an effort to reduce the risk of those complications in the future. Unfortunately, only 43.7% of patients with hypertension have controlled BP.[34] What's more, despite thousands of research studies on hypertension and dozens of readily available and inexpensive medications, that rate has gotten worse over the past 20 years.[34] Given that we know how to treat hypertension, and given what a driver it is of serious disease and death, controlling BP is an obvious and major focus of quality improvement.

So how do we make improvements? Lots of things can contribute to poor BP control, like bad diet, lack of exercise, smoking, lack of insurance, stress, and inability to afford medications. Many of these are quite difficult for a doctor or health system to impact. One area of focus is the current system of "episodic" care, that is, changes in medications or counseling given only at doctor's visits every so often, even though hypertension is a continuous issue. Some managed care plans, like Kaiser Permanente, have moved beyond episodic care by employing teams (such as nurses, pharmacists, and community health workers) to check in on patients frequently and tinker with medications as necessary (ie, the "population health" approach, see Chapter 1). With this new approach, and close attention to quality improvement methods, Kaiser has seen significantly greater improvement in BP control than the rest of the population, as shown in Table 4.2.[35] Value-based care models aim to replicate this success, incentivizing doctors and health systems to improve BP control for their patients.

Disparities and Equity

It's important to think not only about our success in managing a particular priority such as hypertension or cancer screenings but also how that success might differ among groups of people—that is, disparities in care. There are many lenses through which to look at disparities, including age, geographic location, insurance type, gender, race/ethnicity, language, disability,

Table 4.2 Percentage of People With Controlled Blood Pressure, by Population, 2001-2018

	Kaiser—N. California (%)	U.S. HMOs (%)[a]	U.S. population (%)[b]
2018	83[c]	61.3	43.7
2009	80.4[d]	64.1	53
2001	43.6[d]	51.5	34.9

[a]NCQA. Controlling high blood pressure (CBP). https://www.ncqa.org/hedis/measures/controlling-high-blood-pressure/

[b]Muntner P, Hardy ST, Fine LJ, et al. Trends in blood pressure control among US adults with hypertension, 1999-2000 to 2017-2018. *JAMA*. 2020;324(12):1190-1200. doi:10.1001/jama.2020.14545

[c]Permanente Medicine. Kaiser Permanente nation's best at controlling high blood pressure. Published December 6, 2018. https://permanente.org/kaiser-permanente-nations-best-at-controlling-high-blood-pressure/

[d]Jaffe MG, Lee GA, Young JD, Sidney S, Go AS. Improved blood pressure control associated with a large-scale hypertension program. *JAMA*. 2013;310(7):699-705. doi:10.1001/jama.2013.108769

education attainment, and income. As an example, let's zoom out to the big picture: life expectancy. The average life expectancy in the New Orleans metro area is 76.6,[36] which just about matches the national life expectancy of 77.[37] However, if you break down life expectancy for each of the parishes in New Orleans—neighborhoods that are highly segregated by race and income— then you'll find a shocking range in life expectancy, as shown in Figure 4.3. The average might look good, but in fact it is hiding pockets of far worse health outcomes. Addressing disparities is an essential element of improving quality beyond the average. To do so, we need to consider disparities in terms of who develops—or develops worse—disease (ie, societal factors) as well as disparities in the care the medical system provides (ie, medical system factors).[38]

For an example of how averages hide pockets of worse outcomes—and thus worse quality—let's look back at our example of hypertension management from the prior page. We told you that 43.7% of people with hypertension

Life Expectancy by Neighborhood, New Orleans

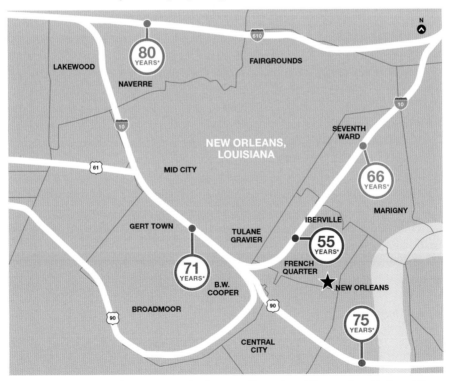

Figure 4.3 Adapted from Centers for Disease Control and Prevention. National Center for Health Statistics. Life expectancy. Accessed July 2022. https://www.rwjf.org/en/library/infographics/new-orleans-map.html

have an optimally controlled BP. But what that statistic is hiding is that non-Hispanic Whites have 7% better control than non-Hispanic Blacks, that those who went to college have 12% better control than those who didn't finish high school, and that those with private insurance have 7% better control than those on Medicaid.[34] Although a quality improvement program aimed at improving overall hypertension control may not be able to address every societal contributor to these disparities, they can still focus their attention and tailor their interventions to address what is modifiable. For instance, the previous section tells us about Kaiser Permanente's improvement in hypertension control in the past 20 years: Kaiser also managed to cut the disparity gap between White and Black patients in half.[39] Any equitable, successful approach to quality improvement must take disparities into account.

In this section, you have reviewed some of the major concepts, processes, and areas of quality improvement. All of this work depends heavily on information technology and EHRs. So let's take a turn toward these fields.

Health Information Technology and Digital Health

In the past decade, U.S. health care made the transition from paper to a digital world (well, not totally … we've kept the pagers and fax machines). This digital transformation has fixed many problems, created new ones, and spawned a huge new field of business and research. The concept of health IT is simple: the application of digital systems to organizing and using health data, from writing prescriptions to transmitting test results digitally to tracking large-scale data trends. However, as with many aspects of health care, this simple concept quickly becomes extremely complicated when put into practice. At its most basic level, health IT refers to EHRs or electronic medical records (EMRs)—systems for charting, coding, and prescribing electronically—but it also encompasses telemedicine, the exchange of health information across systems, and tools designed to help providers avoid mistakes and make the best diagnostic decisions.

In general, you can think of health IT as the use of technology not just to make health care more efficient and less error prone, but rather—on a grander scale—to transform the way that we do business to make delivery of care better and more effective.

Electronic Health Records/Electronic Medical Records

When society upgraded from writing by hand on paper to typing on a computer, we didn't just replicate words in a digital format; we also gained functionality beyond the capabilities of paper—like spellcheck, or the ability to easily reproduce many copies. The same goes for the EHR, which is a digital version of patient charts. The EHR contains the same elements of paper charts (ie, notes, lab values, flowsheets, physician orders) along with elements beyond it (ie, alerts, easy data collection, and messaging to patients). It is not just a record of clinical care; it is also the tool used to get that clinical work done. Further, the EHR is also much harder—and more expensive—to change than a paper form. Thus, although the EHR has opened new possibilities for medical care, its limitations are starkly obvious for all who use it.

The roots of the EHR go way back. The very earliest forms were developed in the 1960s, and, in the 1990s, the Veterans Affairs (VA) was at the forefront of EHR use with home-grown, cutting-edge software.[40] (That no-longer-cutting-edge software is still being used in 2023.[g]) Yet, despite the growth of computerized technology and vendor options, widespread EHR use in nonfederal hospitals didn't occur until after 2009, when the Health Information Technology for Economic and Clinical Health (HITECH) Act was passed by Congress. HITECH incentivized the "meaningful use"[h] of EHRs, and the percentage of hospitals using an EHR went from 10% to 97% in the ensuing 5 years.[41,42]

As of 2021, there are many options for EHRs, but a few vendors dominate the market. The leaders in the inpatient and outpatient settings are mentioned in Table 4.3.

What does an EHR do? It both stores health information as well as forms the processes by which care is provided. If a clinic's or hospital's computer

Table 4.3 EHR Vendor Leaders in Inpatient and Outpatient Settings, 2021

EHR vendor	Market share, 2020 (%)
Epic	31
Cerner	25
Meditech	16
Allscripts	5

EHR, electronic health record. Source: Adapted from Drees J. EHR market share 2021: 10 things to know about major players Epic, Cerner, Meditech & Allscripts. *Becker's Health IT*. Published May 21, 2021. https://www.beckershospitalreview.com/ehrs/ehr-market-share-2021-10-things-to-know-about-major-players-epic-cerner-meditech-allscripts.html

---

[g]Though not for long, as in 2018 the Veterans Health Administration (VHA) announced they would spend $16 billion to switch to Cerner. The first VA, in Washington, transitioned in 2020, with many bumps. This is a fascinating process to watch, connecting technology, difficulties in how systems work and change, and the business of medicine.
[h]Now called the Medicare EHR Incentive Program.

system went down, not only would you not be able to look anything up—you would suddenly lose your process for doing any work. The major functions of the EHR include:

1. **Clinical Documentation ("Notes"):** From clinicians to nurses to physical therapists to social workers, from documenting an operation to documenting a simple phone call.

2. **Computerized Physician Order Entry:** Allows providers to prescribe medications, order tests, and give other types of instructions electronically—both in and out of the hospital. Eighty-four percent of outpatient prescribers send prescriptions electronically to pharmacies.[43,i] In the hospital, the EHR also tracks medication administration by pharmacies and nurses.

3. **Test Results:** Any user can see all historical results from their system (so the clinician can look up the result of a colonoscopy from 7 years ago), as well as use functions like graphing test results over time.

4. **Patient Portals:** Increasingly, EHRs have included a way for patients to see their test results, request and even schedule appointments, and send messages to their care team. As of 2021, some of this is even required by law: the 21st century Cures Act bans "information blocking," meaning health systems need to share data with patients in real time.[44]

All of the above is true, but for someone who has actually used an EHR, it might paint an overly rosy picture. The information in EHRs is often incredibly fragmented and can be time consuming and difficult to navigate, with a design more like a messy filing cabinet than a seamless digital work platform.

Health Informatics

Health informatics analyzes data from EMRs and other sources to improve the delivery of care through a variety of methods. Clinical informatics encompasses many elements of both operations (ie, the practical aspects of how care gets delivered) and research (ie, how we can learn from data).

One major way for informatics to improve care is through clinical decision support (CDS). CDS can help with decisions about medication prescribing,

---

[i]Interestingly, even as electronic prescribing ("e-Rx") became widespread, the *cancellation* of prescriptions did not. Many doctors assumed that deleting a medication in the system would notify the pharmacy, just as prescribing did, but this was not the case: up to 5% of canceled medications were still dispensed. Instead, technology vendors charged extra for the additional functionality of "e-cancel Rx." This is obviously a major issue for quality in medication reconciliation, and an interesting one for thinking through how the business of medicine affects delivery (https://jamanetwork-com.ucsf.idm.oclc.org/journals/jamainternalmedicine/fullarticle/2783454).

adherence to guidelines, and making diagnoses. A simple CDS tool can check a prescribed medication against patient data such as allergies, renal function, and other medications, then display this information to the prescribing clinician in real time. This can both save the prescriber time, as well as ensure this kind of check doesn't get forgotten. You can probably imagine how a CDS tool might be designed to help prevent central line bloodstream infections, for example, by alerting medical teams to how long a central line has been in place.

Some other examples of basic informatics projects you'd find in any health system include:

- An order set including all the lab tests and referrals that might be necessary for treating a patient with diabetes
- Dashboard for primary care providers showing rates of cancer screening among different patient groups
- Visual display showing timing of blood product transfusions along with hemoglobin and coagulation levels to help assess response and inform decision-making
- Tracking system for patient outreach efforts for vaccinations, to identify and follow up with patients who did not respond
- Decision support and recommendations for ordering guideline-appropriate imaging tests

Again, these are basic projects, and many systems boast much more impressive examples. However, the landscape of informatics innovations is uneven (as is regulation). A single institution might have quite sophisticated data capabilities in some areas yet still struggle with one of the basic projects above.

Interoperability and Health Information Exchange

Here's a common story: A patient moves across the country and gets a new primary care clinician. The new clinician would like to review their old records, but the patient has been seen in about five different clinics and four different health systems in the past 10 years. The patient has to remember where they got care, they have to sign a release of information for each place, and the new clinic has to request the records. A few weeks later, and if everything goes right, the fax machine spits out 250 pages for the new clinician to sift through. Here's another common story: a patient switches to a clinic down the street, and the same thing happens.

Near or far, the EHRs in our example aren't sharing information. Interoperability is the technical ability for two different electronic systems to communicate data, and Health Information Exchange (HIE) is the actual sharing of that data. Mostly, data sharing is accomplished through application programming interfaces (APIs), which are the same technology that allows you to share data among apps, though in this case the APIs must meet federal regulations set by the Office of the National Coordinator.

Interoperability is also sometimes simply called data sharing, and anything opposed to it is called information blocking. If our new clinician can see information about her patient from outside her own organization in a standardized format then she is in a better position to make diagnosis and treatment decisions. Data sharing is a major goal of health IT as well as health systems, as a step toward increasing efficiency, improving patient transfers, decreasing repeated tests, and ensuring clinical teams have the right information at the right time. But even the goal of information alignment still isn't perfectly aligned: there are about 100 separate HIE organizations! The largest umbrella organization is the Strategic Health Information Exchange Collaborative, a "network of networks" representing over 90% of the U.S. population.[45]

But data sharing is not easy. Barriers come from the health system side (fears of making it easier for patients to switch to competitor health systems) and the EHR vendor side (fears of losing proprietary information or making it easier for health systems to switch to competitor vendors). The federal government has stepped in, with the 21st century Cures Act, to define and penalize information blocking behaviors by EHRs and health systems. As of 2023, significant progress has been made, but surveys of HIEs reported that information blocking remains common, most often in the form of EHR vendors charging high prices for interoperability functions.[46] That being said, there is a lot of energy in this area—particularly with Fast Healthcare Interoperability Resources (FHIR, pronounced "fire")[47]—and this section is sure to go out-of-date quickly.

Patient Access and Portals

Information blocking applies to patients, too, many of whom have for years fought to have better access to their own records. Although federal and state laws have long required hospitals and clinics to provide their records upon request, in practice this has been cumbersome and expensive for patients. (One study with "secret shopper" record requests found a hospital charging $500 for 200 pages of the patient's own information![48])

A patient portal is a secure website giving patients digital access to portions of their personal health information as well as allowing actions such as messaging their doctors, requesting refills, and completing forms. The very first patient portals were developed in the late 1990s.[49] After the HITECH Act in 2009, most health systems offered a patient portal, but not that many patients used them—until the COVID-19 pandemic. The pandemic, by limiting in-person care, incentivized patients to activate their portal accounts and health systems to make the portals more user-friendly (ie, adding self-scheduling tools).[50] As of 2021, federal law also requires that all results and notes be available in real time electronically through patient portals. This is frequently referred to as "open notes" and was a long-term objective of advocacy groups.[51]

As useful as access to one's notes is, it's important to keep equity in mind. There are concerns that the growth of online tools and telehealth will increase access only for some patients, and in fact will worsen disparities in care for patients without reliable internet access, without computers, and with low digital literacy.

It's also important to keep in mind that although the ability to message or send data to a clinician outside of visits is convenient for patients and probably better for their care, answering messages (which have increased dramatically since 2020) and reviewing data are still (unpaid) work for clinicians, because reimbursement and delivery (including much of the quality improvement system) are still structured almost entirely around episodic office visits. There are some efforts to reimburse for this work (like at the University of California San Francisco[52]), but for now this is an example in which technology has outpaced delivery.

Data Analytics

How many patients in a primary care clinic have uncontrolled BP? When medical information like BP was written on paper in individual charts, answering that question meant a time-consuming and cumbersome process of physically flipping through charts; now, you can pull BP readings from thousands of patients in a health system in 3 minutes. By putting medical charts into an electronic format, health IT has essentially "created" large amounts of data. The EHR contains information far beyond BP, including demographics, social determinants, lab values, hospitalizations, diagnoses, prescriptions, and spending. Data analytics investigates what that data can tell us.

This is often at the level of a clinic or institution, perhaps in quality improvement or population health management efforts. For instance, a primary care clinic might use data analytics to track their success at controlling their patients' BP, to find subgroups that have worse control, and to show physicians how they compare to each other. A population health team might extend that effort to dozens of clinics and thousands of patients in a health care network.

On a large scale, sometimes representing millions of patients, data analytics holds further promise on how we address health and delivery of care. Large datasets can be analyzed to discover patterns, make connections between seemingly unconnected factors, and learn how to predict and solve problems. A simple way of using data analytics might be predicting who won't show up for appointments. A complex way might be to predict who will get breast cancer. See Section "Where Are We Headed With Health IT?" in this chapter to consider some ways in which big data might transform health care.

Beyond the promises of improved health, large datasets are also used to improve finances. An insurance company uses data to figure out which providers overbill so they can cut those providers out of their network or negotiate lower reimbursements. A pharmaceutical company uses data on prescribing patterns to target which providers to market to. A hospital uses data to determine which of their services are being denied, and how to improve reimbursement.

(This may prompt the question: who owns all this data? You have a right to your health data, but you do not "own" it, in the legal sense. Deidentified patient datasets are often sold by health care organizations. In 2022, IBM Watson Health closed up most of its data analytics shop and sold its health data to a private equity firm for $1 billion, just 6 years after it launched with a goal of using big data to transform cancer care.[53])

Information Overload

Health IT has done a great job of making mountains of data available. It's done a not-so-great job of organizing that data. It takes time to review all that information and find what you need, especially if you've got to look at 20 different places in the computer to find it, and then you have to summarize it all. In the clinic, nearly a third of a doctor's time per patient is spent on reviewing data ("chart review").[54] In the hospital, internal medicine residents spend 43% of their time on the medical record (and only 13% face-to-face with patients).[55] Sometimes that mountain of data feels like an avalanche.

Electronic notes can worsen the overload with "note bloat." In writing a medical note, the EHR offers templates, canned phrases, and even the ability to just copy forward and update an old note. With these tools, notes have gotten longer and longer, with less and less useful information in them.[j] Ask any doctor about note bloat, and they'll rant about getting faxed notes that are just eight pages of templated text with an out-of-date exam and little if any useful clue as to what the other doctor was thinking … then ask that same doctor if they use templates and copy/paste, too (the answer will be yes).

Furthermore, even safety alerts meant to be helpful can become part of the problem. Unless alerts are calibrated to pop up only when appropriate, users can become jaded about their utility and just "click through" without paying attention, that is, "alert fatigue." Fatigue isn't surprising when, for example, intensive care unit (ICU) physicians see over 150 EHR alerts per

---

[j]It is important to note that a lot of the bloat isn't because of the tools themselves but rather because of the extensive compliance and reimbursement requirements for clinical documentation.

patient per day, many irrelevant.[56] Studies show that clinicians are less likely to pay attention to alerts the more often they receive them.[57]

Finally, there's the flip side: because analysis of a dataset is only as good as the data in it, a lot depends on clinicians and clinical staff to enter information—and to enter it the right way. This can happen in little ways, say, clinicians who have to enter their patients' home BPs so they get "counted" for the metrics. It can also occur in large ways, say, clinicians who accidentally but systematically miscode a condition, so that we don't know the actual prevalence of the disease. In both cases, actual care of the patients is unaffected. This can leave clinicians feeling like data entry clerks.

Information overload can contribute to burnout (see Section "EHRs and Burnout" later in this chapter) and it underscores the importance of not just shifting the medical record to a digital format, but rather of truly understanding the workflow of health care workers and using *well-designed* technology to augment it.

Cybersecurity

Unfortunately, moving everything online and to networks (both the information itself as well as the actual operations of how things get done) leaves health systems vulnerable to cyberattacks.

These cyberattacks, usually in the form of ransomware, have been on the rise since the COVID-19 pandemic. In 2020, 92 attacks affected 600 health care organizations and 18 million patients, adding to the 25 million patient records affected in the prior 4 years.[58] Globally, one in three hospitals reported a cyberattack of some sort.[59] Although ransom demands themselves may be relatively low (organizations are encouraged not to pay, but many still do), the inability to perform regular clinical operations during the attack leads to major loss of revenue.

More importantly, these attacks threaten patient privacy as well as safety. The first patient death attributable to a ransomware attack may have occurred in 2019, when decreased computer monitoring (because of computers being down in the attack) at an Alabama hospital was implicated in the death of a newborn.[60]

Where Are We Headed With Health IT?

In this section more than any other, this book is already out-of-date. Like the rest of the tech world, health-related technologies are advancing incredibly quickly. Some areas already in development, and which we expect to see blossom, include:

- **Tracking Data From Patient Devices:** Currently, about 21% of adults report wearing a smart fitness tracker of some sort, though interoperability and privacy concerns still limit the integration of this data into EHRs.[61] Wearable or personal health technology will grow as a field and in many cases will expand and transform how we deliver care. For instance, continuous glucose monitors (as opposed to intermittent fingerstick glucometers) are already changing how we think about diabetes monitoring and treatment.

- **Using Artificial Intelligence (AI) to Offload Some Clinical Tasks:** Radiology has seen the biggest growth in AI, with many studies comparing AI to physicians in terms of rating scans as normal or not.[62] Although AI is unlikely to completely displace clinicians, it is likely to become an integral part of how clinicians deliver care, particularly in fields involving images or large amounts of data.

- **Using Big Data to Predict and Prevent Illness:** There are already efforts to use machine learning to predict in-hospital mortality,[63] mostly focused on infection.[64] In the future, big data could be used to predict all kinds of adverse health events (falls, cancers, bed sores, etc).

We are likely to see amazing advancements in care because of ever-progressing technology. However, we would be wise to remember that difficult problems in medicine are just that—difficult. How much does wearable technology matter to a patient who cannot afford to go see his physician? What does machine learning do for a patient who cannot understand her prescription instructions because they are written in a language she doesn't speak? Slick technology may be cool, but it doesn't fix the system. If health IT is to see its promise, it will require good old-fashioned understanding of human behavior and good design alongside digital innovations.

Issues

At the beginning of this chapter, we acknowledged that, at first glance, quality and technology might not feel like connected topics. Even as you've read through the disparate and wide-ranging details within this chapter, we hope you see the connecting thread of how these fields have revolutionized the way health care works. Assessing quality of care relies heavily on the data collection and analytic capabilities of health IT. Similarly, digital innovations cannot be assumed to improve quality; digital health should be assessed for its impact on outcomes and disparities just like any other element of care.

Another connecting thread of these topics is that both have had significant unintended consequences. Let's talk through two major concerns for clinicians and health systems.

Choosing the Right Metrics

We can all agree on the desire to improve quality of care, but how to do so is another matter. Efforts to improve quality combine policymaking, research, HIT, and reimbursement to change the way care is delivered (essentially tying together all the chapters of this book).

But the devil is in choosing what to measure, how to define and track changes, and predicting and mitigating unintended consequences. One high-profile example of questionable quality improvement involves a policy effort to improve sepsis mortality. Sepsis is when infection causes an overwhelming inflammatory response in the body, which itself causes damage to organs and tissues. Sepsis is expensive, has a high mortality rate, and is treatable, making its treatment a good measure for policymakers to use to compare hospital quality and incentivize improvement. In 2015, Medicare instituted a performance measure called SEP-1, which focused on requiring a specific "bundle" of tests and treatments, and used the metric of how often this bundle was used to compare hospitals in the Hospital Compare website. But many felt that the metric had been rushed based on not-yet-established data, and SEP-1 had to be revised for elements lacking in scientific basis.[65] Ultimately, the SEP-1 bundle—as well as many of the tools used to institute it, such as EHR alerts—hasn't been shown to clearly improve sepsis treatment and mortality. Critics feel that these policies led to too much energy spent on documentation, on labeling even the mildest of cases (who would have survived anyway) as sepsis, and on demonstrating compliance rather than on actually improving care of the sickest patients.

In addition, there can be other unintended consequences to metrics. For instance, a New York quality scorecard for coronary artery bypass surgery *did* lead to an improvement in mortality for this procedure in the 1990s. However, surgeons expressed greater reluctance to perform the procedure on their sickest patients (who were more likely to die regardless), and more frequently transferred them out of state to get the procedure elsewhere.[66] Nearly 90% of interventional cardiologists think the public reporting of physician-specific mortality statistics leads to some patients not receiving a procedure they might benefit from.[67] With metrics, you can look better by doing better, but you can also look "better" by shifting who gets included in the numbers (called cherry-picking).

A principle of quality improvement is "if you can't measure it, you can't improve it." Yet, as Jerry Z. Muller writes in *The Tyranny of Metrics*,

> Not everything that is important is measurable, and much that is measurable is not important. Many jobs have multiple facets, and measuring only a few aspects creates incentives to neglect the rest. When organizations committed to metrics wake up to this fact, they

typically add more performance measures—which creates a cascade of data, data that becomes ever less useful, while gathering it sucks up more and more time and resources.[68]

Although no one is suggesting there should be *no* quality metrics—they really are necessary!—many do emphasize that metrics should be chosen carefully, based on high-quality evidence, and with follow-up studies to demonstrate the efficacy of the metrics themselves.

EHRs and Burnout

Who could argue against CPOE, which eliminates handwriting errors, and CDS, which can flag dangerous drug interactions? What clinician is unhappy about checking a computer for a test result rather than running across the hospital flipping through charts all day? What patient is upset that their information is available 24/7 in a portal? EHRs have changed health care for the better, and they're here to stay. But not all of the changes have been good.

Switching to an EHR from a paper charting system takes a lot of money (we mean a *lot* of money, estimated at $15,000 to $70,000 per provider—meaning billions for a large hospital system[69]), in addition to time training and lost efficiency as providers learn the new system, so the outcomes better be worth the investment. We can think of the outcomes in two buckets: first, clinical care and patient outcomes. Second, job satisfaction for the health care workers who have to use the EHR.

In terms of patient outcomes, the evidence is mixed. Large studies looking at quality differences between hospitals with and without full EHR adoption, mostly conducted between 2005 and 2015, generally found no effect in overall patient outcomes.[70-73] Although writing this in 2022, nearly all health systems have fully implemented EHRs, so it would be difficult to run further comparative studies. It seems likely that EHRs have made a big difference in data tracking and quality improvement in many specific areas, such as CLABSI. An emerging question, at this point, is how the design and usability of the EHR itself affects quality of care.

In terms of job satisfaction, EHRs get a lot of blame. Anyone who uses an EHR (provider, nurse, social worker, medical assistant, etc) will tell you that EHRs are not designed to prioritize clinical workflows. Physician wellness advocate Dr Christine Sinsky describes it taking 32 clicks in her EHR just to document giving a flu shot.[74] Time-motion studies show that resident physicians spend more time on the EHR than they do with patients, both in the hospital[55] as well as in the primary care clinic.[75] Physicians who self-report burnout in surveys frequently point to the EHR, and one study found that more after-hours time on the EHR as well as higher EHR message volume were independently predictive of emotional exhaustion.[76] It can feel like death by a thousand clicks.

From a big picture perspective, we cannot blame EHRs for everything. The fact that they haven't revolutionized quality and safety outcomes reflects the importance of culture and behavior change. And the fact that EHRs contribute to burnout also reflects their use to enforce onerous documentation requirements for compliance, reimbursement, and quality metrics—in many cases, these requirements themselves are the problem, not the computers. EHRs can and should be improved (it shouldn't take 32 clicks to report that you gave a flu shot!), but so should the system in which they are used.

Safety and Medical Malpractice: With Brian Yagi

In this chapter, we've discussed the ways that health care organizations work internally to improve the quality and safety of their care, but this isn't the only way. Patient safety can also be addressed outside the medical system—in the courts, called medical malpractice. In contrast to the systems-focused methods we've discussed so far, medical malpractice focuses on the harm done to a small subset of patients because of error by individual providers.

Patients who believe they have been injured in some way by a health care provider can file a medical malpractice claim. To prove malpractice, the patient must show both that they were harmed as well as that the harm was caused by the provider's negligence, meaning that the provider didn't practice medicine consistent with the accepted standard of care. If a patient wins a case or a favorable settlement, the health care provider may have to compensate the patient for loss of income because of injury and for noneconomic losses, such as pain and suffering. The idea is that error itself imposes cost, and malpractice lawsuits shift that cost from patients (ie, victims of error) to providers (ie, perpetrators of error). The threat or reality of high malpractice costs should ideally force providers and systems to improve their unsafe behaviors. Although most malpractice claims are made against physicians, claims can be brought against any health care clinician, including students. To protect against the financial risk of future malpractice lawsuits, most physicians purchase malpractice insurance.

A few key facts about medical malpractice:

- The overwhelming majority of patients who receive negligent care don't file malpractice claims (Figure 4.4).[60]
- Only one-fifth of malpractice claims result in payment to the patient; the average payment is $365,503. However, proving that there's no liability isn't cheap for physicians either—averaging $191,341 for a successful trial

defense, and $30,000 even if the claim is dropped, withdrawn, or dismissed before making it to the court room.[77]

■ Malpractice claims and payments have decreased significantly over the past 20 years. The number of paid claims nationwide decreased by half from 1992 to 2016.[78]

■ By the time they reach age 55, nearly half of physicians will have been sued for malpractice.[77] But only 1% of physicians account for a third of all paid malpractice claims.[79,k]

■ The cost of malpractice insurance varies dramatically by location and specialty. Premiums for a general internist in Maryland run around $7,000 per year, whereas those for neurosurgeons in Long Island, NY, cost $330,000 or more.[80,81]

Financial costs of medical malpractice were rising precipitously in the early 1990s. This, in turn, led to higher malpractice insurance rates for providers and in turn to a number of states passing laws aimed at curbing medical malpractice lawsuits. These laws, collectively called "tort reform," were passed in 33 states and include provisions that limit the amount of noneconomic damages (ie, pain and suffering) that injured plaintiffs can recover. Some states also created more procedural hurdles for plaintiffs, such as requiring them to have an expert witness review the facts before a lawsuit is even filed.[82] Some institutions require arbitration agreements, which can limit damages, as well. States that passed tort reform laws saw a significant decline in the total number of malpractice cases, and this effect persisted after a few of the states attempted to reverse their tort reform laws.[83]

The fear of litigation has also caused a shift in the way that physicians provide care to patients, which is known as "defensive medicine." There are two types of defensive medicine: positive, in which physicians overuse services to "cover their bases" in case of a lawsuit, rather than to practice evidence-based, cost-effective medicine (one of many drivers of low-value care, see Section "Why Does U.S. Health Care Cost So Much?" in Chapter 3); and negative, in which physicians avoid high-risk patients and procedures they fear could be a higher risk for litigation. This isn't just a theoretical problem—in surveys, more than four out of five specialist physicians report practicing positive defensive medicine.[63,64] Defenders of the system, though, would counter that as long as providers adhere to the standard of care, low-value care or "defensive medicine" is not necessary to protect a provider from malpractice liability.

When patients have suffered harm because of medical care, we have two goals: (1) to compensate victims of poor medical care, and (2) to reduce error

---

[k]Individual bad providers can be reported to state medical boards, although they may be allowed to continue practicing.

Below the Iceberg: Medical Errors as Compared to Medical Malpractice

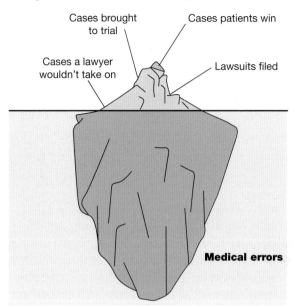

Figure 4.4

to prevent harm to future patients. The current medical malpractice approach may not be the best system to advance these goals, and tort reform focused on reducing the costs associated with goal #1 without addressing or advancing goal #2 (reduce error). In fact, there's evidence that risk of malpractice liability does not improve health care quality at all.[84]

Alternatives to the current malpractice system are gaining interest across the country. Many institutions now openly disclose medical errors to injured patients and offer a settlement up-front. If the injured party accepts the settlement offer, they sign away their right to bring the case as a civil suit or tort. The University of Michigan is an example of an early adopter of the "disclose and offer" system, and it saw a significant decline in the number of claims filed by patients as well as total costs of addressing malpractice claims.[85] Another alternative is to decouple harm from negligence and to compensate patients who experienced harm through a "no-fault" system. In the United States, examples include the National Vaccine Injury Compensation Program, which provides financial repayments to people who have a serious adverse reaction to a recommended vaccine, as well as Worker's Compensation, which provides financial and medical benefits to workers who are injured or become ill on the job. Such no-fault compensation systems exist for medical harm in other countries, such as New Zealand and Sweden.[86]

References

1. Donaldson MS, Corrigan JM, Kohn LT, eds. *To Err Is Human: Building a Safer Health System.* National Academies Press; 2000.

2. Bates DW, Singh H. Two decades since to err is human: an assessment of progress and emerging priorities in patient safety. *Health Aff (Millwood).* 2018;37(11):1736-1743. doi:10.1377/hlthaff.2018.0738

3. Mitchell PH. Defining patient safety and quality care. In: Hughes RG, ed. *Patient Safety and Quality: An Evidence-Based Handbook for Nurses.* Agency for Healthcare Research and Quality (US); 2008. https://www.ncbi.nlm.nih.gov/books/NBK2681/

4. Institute of Medicine (US) Committee on Quality of Health Care in America. Improving the 21st-century health care system. *Crossing the Quality Chasm: A New Health System for the 21st Century.* National Academies Press (US); 2001. https://www.ncbi.nlm.nih.gov/books/NBK222265/

5. Institute for Healthcare Improvement. IHI triple aim initiative. Published July 2022. http://www.ihi.org/Engage/Initiatives/TripleAim/Pages/default.aspx

6. Woolf SH, Schoomaker H. Life expectancy and mortality rates in the United States, 1959-2017. *JAMA.* 2019;322(20):1996-2016. doi:10.1001/jama.2019.16932

7. McGlynn EA, Asch SM, Adams J, et al. The quality of health care delivered to adults in the United States. *N Engl J Med.* 2003;348(26):2635-2645. doi:10.1056/NEJMsa022615

8. Russell TA, Fritschel E, Do J, et al. Minimizing central line-associated bloodstream infections in a high-acuity liver transplant intensive care unit. *Am J Infect Control.* 2019;47(3):305-312. doi:10.1016/j.ajic.2018.08.006

9. Centers for Disease Control and Prevention. Vital signs: central line—associated blood stream infections—United States, 2001, 2008, and 2009. *Morbid Mortal Wkly Rep.* 2011;60(08):243-248. https://www.cdc.gov/mmwr/preview/mmwrhtml/mm6008a4.htm

10. Centers for Disease Control and Prevention. Healthcare- and community-associated infections. Published July 2022. https://arpsp.cdc.gov/profile/infections/

11. Leape L. The checklist conundrum. *N Engl J Med.* 2014;370:1063-1064.

12. Agency for Healthcare Research and Quality. About learning health systems. Accessed July 2022. https://www.ahrq.gov/learning-health-systems/about.html

13. Wadhera RK, Figueroa JF, Joynt Maddox KE, Rosenbaum LS, Kazi DS, Yeh RW. Quality measure development and associated spending by the Centers for Medicare & Medicaid Services. *JAMA.* 2020;323(16):1614-1616. doi:10.1001/jama.2020.1816

14. Casalino LP, Gans D, Weber R, et al. US physician practices spend more than $15.4 billion annually to report quality measures. *Health Aff (Millwood).* 2016;35(3):401-406. doi:10.1377/hlthaff.2015.1258

15. Joszt L. The evolution of quality measurement and efforts to streamline reporting. *Am J Manag Care.* Published July 17, 2018. https://www.ajmc.com/view/the-evolution-of-quality-measurement-and-efforts-to-streamline-reporting

16. Table: 33 ACO Quality Measures. July 2022. https://www.cms.gov/medicare/medicare-fee-for-service-payment/sharedsavingsprogram/downloads/aco-shared-savings-program-quality-measures.pdf

17. SingleCare. Journal of Community Hospital Internal Medicine Perspectives, 2016. NCBI, 2019. https://www.singlecare.com/blog/news/medication-errors-statistics/

18. Health.gov. National action plan for ADE prevention. Office of Disease Prevention and Health Promotion (ODPHP). 2022. https://health.gov/our-work/national-health-initiatives/health-care-quality/adverse-drug-events

19. Patient Safety Network (PSNet). Medication errors and adverse drug events. Published September 7, 2019. https://psnet.ahrq.gov/primer/medication-errors-and-adverse-drug-events

20. Choi I, Lee SM, Flynn L, et al. Incidence and treatment costs attributable to medication errors in hospitalized patients. *Res Social Adm Pharm.* 2016;12(3):428-437. doi:10.1016/j.sapharm.2015.08.006

21. Evidence Report/Technology Assessment. Number 211. Making health care safer II: an updated critical analysis of the evidence for patient safety practices. Prepared by RAND Corporation. Prepared for Agency for Healthcare Research and Quality, U.S. Department of Health and Human Services. AHRQ Publication No. 13-E001-EF. Published March 2013. https://www.ahrq.gov/sites/default/files/wysiwyg/research/findings/evidence-based-reports/services/quality/patientsftyupdate/ptsafetyII-full.pdf

22. Laurance J. Peter Pronovost: champion of checklists in critical care. *Lancet.* 2009;374(9688):443. doi:10.1016/S0140-6736(09)61439-2. https://www.sciencedirect.com/science/article/pii/S0140673609614392

23. Centers for Disease Control and Prevention. Healthcare-Associated Infections (HAIs). https://www.cdc.gov/hai/data/index.html

24. CMS.gov. Hospital-acquired conditions. July 2022. https://www.cms.gov/Medicare/Medicare-Fee-for-Service-Payment/HospitalAcqCond/Hospital-Acquired_Conditions

25. Vidyarthi AR, Arora V, Schnipper JL, et al. Managing discontinuity in academic medical centers: strategies for a safe and effective resident sign-out. *J Hosp Med.* 2006;1(4):257-266.

26. Clarke M. I-PASS and SBAR handoff tools have proven benefits. *Patient Safety & Quality Healthcare (PSQH).* Published April 13, 2016. https://www.psqh.com/news/i-pass-and-sbar-handoff-tools-have-proven-benefits/

27. Forster AJ, Murff HJ, Peterson JF, Gandhi TK, Bates DW. The incidence and severity of adverse events affecting patients after discharge from the hospital. *Ann Intern Med.* 2003;138(3):161-167. doi:10.7326/0003-4819-138-3-200302040-00007

28. Kim CS, Flanders SA. In the clinic. Transitions of care. *Ann Intern Med.* 2013;158(5 Pt 1):ITC3-1. doi:10.7326/0003-4819-158-5-201303050-01003

29. Levine DM, Linder JA, Landon BE. The quality of outpatient care delivered to adults in the United States, 2002 to 2013. *JAMA Intern Med.* 2016;176(12):1778-1790. doi:10.1001/jamainternmed.2016.6217

30. Borsky A, Zhan C, Miller T, et al. Few Americans receive all high-priority, appropriate clinical preventive services. *Health Aff (Millwood).* 2018;37(6):925-928. doi:10.1377/hlthaff.2017.1248

31. Centers for Disease Control and Prevention. Sharp declines in breast and cervical cancer screening. Published June 30, 2021. https://www.cdc.gov/media/releases/2021/p0630-cancer-screenings.html

32. Office of Disease Prevention and Health Promotion. Clinical preventive services. https://www.healthypeople.gov/2020/leading-health-indicators/2020-lhi-topics/Clinical-Preventive-Services/data

33. Centers for Disease Control and Prevention. Hypertension. July 2022. https://www.cdc.gov/nchs/fastats/hypertension.htm

34. Muntner P, Hardy ST, Fine LJ, et al. Trends in blood pressure control among US adults with hypertension, 1999-2000 to 2017-2018. *JAMA*. 2020;324(12):1190-1200. doi:10.1001/jama.2020.14545

35. McGlynn EA. Improving the quality of U.S. health care—what will it take? *N Engl J Med*. 2020;383(9):801-803. doi:10.1056/NEJMp2022644

36. Habans R, Losh J, Weinstein R, Teller A. Placing prosperity: neighborhoods and life expectancy in the New Orleans metro. *The Data Center*. Published August 13, 2020. https://www.datacenterresearch.org/reports_analysis/placing-prosperity/

37. Centers for Disease Control and Prevention. National Center for Health Statistics. Life expectancy. Accessed July 2022. https://www.cdc.gov/nchs/fastats/life-expectancy.htm

38. Metro map: New Orleans, Louisiana—infographic. *Robert Wood Johnson Foundation*. Published June 19, 2013. https://www.rwjf.org/en/library/infographics/new-orleans-map.html

39. Bartolome RE, Chen A, Handler J, Platt ST, Gould B. Population care management and team-based approach to reduce racial disparities among African Americans/Blacks with hypertension. *Perm J*. 2016;20(1):53-59. doi:10.7812/TPP/15-052

40. Atherton J. Development of the electronic health record. *Virtual Mentor*. 2011;13(3):186-189. doi:10.1001/virtualmentor.2011.13.3.mhst1-1103

41. Jha AK, DesRoches CM, Campbell EG, et al. Use of electronic health records in US hospitals. *N Engl J Med*. 2009;360(16):1628-1638.

42. Office of the National Coordinator for Health Information Technology. Non-federal acute care hospital electronic health record adoption. Health IT Quick-Stat #47. Published September 2017. https://www.healthit.gov/data/quickstats/non-federal-acute-care-hospital-electronic-health-record-adoption

43. National Progress Report 2020. Surescripts. https://surescripts.com/news-center/national-progress-report-2020

44. ONC's Cures Act Final Rule supports seamless and secure access, exchange, and use of electronic health information. *ONC's Cures Act Final Rule*. Published July 2022. https://www.healthit.gov/curesrule/

45. SHIEC/America's HIEs. Introducing civitas networks for health. Published July 2022. https://strategichie.com/

46. Everson J, Patel V, Adler-Milstein J. Information blocking remains prevalent at the start of 21st Century Cures Act: results from a survey of health information exchange organizations. *J Am Med Inf Assoc* 2021;28(4):727-732. doi:10.1093/jamia/ocaa323

47. The Office of the National Coordinator for Health Information Technology. What is FHIR®? July 2022. https://www.healthit.gov/sites/default/files/2019-08/ONCFHIRFSWhatIsFHIR.pdf

48. Lye CT, Forman HP, Gao R, et al. Assessment of US hospital compliance with regulations for patients' requests for medical records [published correction appears in *JAMA Netw Open*. 2018 Dec 7;1(8):e186463]. *JAMA Netw Open*. 2018;1(6):e183014. doi:10.1001/jamanetworkopen.2018.3014

49. Halamka JD, Mandl KD, Tang PC. Early experiences with personal health records. *J Am Med Inform Assoc*. 2008;15(1):1-7. doi:10.1197/jamia.M256

50. Johnson C, Richwine C, Patel V. Individuals' access and use of patient portals and smartphone health apps, 2020. ONC Data Brief, No. 57. Office of the National Coordinator for Health Information Technology. Published September 2021.

51. Everyone on the same page. *Open Notes*. Accessed July 2022. https://www.opennotes.org/

52. Ravindranath M. For doctors drowning in emails, one health system's new strategy: pay for replies. STAT. Health Tech. Published January 21, 2022. https://www.statnews.com/2022/01/21/doctors-health-ucsf-patient-emails/

53. Davis MF, Deveau S, Davalos J. IBM sells some Watson Health assets for more than $1 billion. Bloomberg US Edition. Published January 21, 2022. https://www.bloomberg.com/news/articles/2022-01-21/ibm-is-said-to-near-sale-of-watson-health-to-francisco-partners

54. Overhage JM, McCallie D Jr. Physician time spent using the electronic health record during outpatient encounters: a descriptive study [published correction appears in *Ann Intern Med*. 2020 Oct 6;173(7):596]. *Ann Intern Med*. 2020;172(3):169-174. doi:10.7326/M18-3684

55. Chaiyachati KH, Shea JA, Asch DA, et al. Assessment of inpatient time allocation among first-year internal medicine residents using time-motion observations. *JAMA Intern Med*. 2019;179(6):760-767. doi:10.1001/jamainternmed.2019.0095

56. Kizzier-Carnahan V, Artis KA, Mohan V, Gold JA. Frequency of passive EHR alerts in the ICU: another form of alert fatigue? *J Patient Saf*. 2019;15(3):246-250. doi:10.1097/PTS.0000000000000270

57. Ancker JS, Edwards A, Nosal S, et al. Effects of workload, work complexity, and repeated alerts on alert fatigue in a clinical decision support system [published correction appears in *BMC Med Inform Decis Mak*. 2019 Nov 18;19(1):227]. *BMC Med Inform Decis Mak*. 2017;17(1):36. doi:10.1186/s12911-017-0430-8

58. Bischoff P. Ransomware attacks on US healthcare organizations cost $20.8bn in 2020. *Comparitech*. Updated March 10, 2021. https://www.comparitech.com/blog/information-security/ransomware-attacks-hospitals-data/

59. The state of ransomware in healthcare 2021. *A Sophos Whitepaper*. Published May 2021. https://www.sophos.com/en-us/medialibrary/pdfs/whitepaper/sophos-state-of-ransomware-in-healthcare-2021-wp.pdf

60. Poulsen K, McMillan R, Evans M. A hospital hit by hackers, a baby in distress: the case of the first alleged ransomware death. *The Wall Street Journal*. Published September 30, September 2021. https://www.wsj.com/articles/ransomware-hackers-hospital-first-alleged-death-11633008116

61. Vogels EA. About one-in-five Americans use a smart watch or fitness tracker. *Pew Research Center*. Published January 9, 2020. https://www.pewresearch.org/fact-tank/2020/01/09/about-one-in-five-americans-use-a-smart-watch-or-fitness-tracker/

62. Amisha, Malik P, Pathania M, Rathaur VK. Overview of artificial intelligence in medicine. *J Family Med Prim Care*. 2019;8(7):2328-2331. doi:10.4103/jfmpc.jfmpc_440_19

63. Chi S, Guo A, Heard K, et al. Development and structure of an accurate machine learning algorithm to predict inpatient mortality and hospice outcomes in the coronavirus disease 2019 era. *Med Care*. 2022;60(5):381-386. doi:10.1097/MLR.0000000000001699

64. Gelfand A. Warning! Sepsis Ahead: a leading killer of hospitalized patients just may have met its match. *John Hopkins Medicine*. News & Publications. Published Spring/Summer 2021. https://www.hopkinsmedicine.org/news/articles/warning-sepsis-ahead

65. Wang J, Strich JR, Applefeld WN, et al. Driving blind: instituting SEP-1 without high quality outcomes data [published correction appears in *J Thorac Dis*. 2021 Jun;13(6):3932-3933]. *J Thorac Dis*. 2020;12(suppl 1):S22-S36. doi:10.21037/jtd.2019.12.100

66. Werner RM, Asch DA. The unintended consequences of publicly reporting quality information. *JAMA*. 2005;293(10):1239-1244. doi:10.1001/jama.293.10.1239

67. Narins CR, Dozier AM, Ling FS, Zareba W. The influence of public reporting of outcome data on medical decision making by physicians. *Arch Intern Med.* 2005;165(1):83-87. doi:10.1001/archinte.165.1.83

68. Muller JZ. *The Tyranny of Metrics.* Princeton University Press; 2018:17-19.

69. HealthIT.gov. Frequently asked questions. July 2022. https://www.healthit.gov/faq/how-much-going-cost-me

70. Yanamadala S, Morrison D, Curtin C, McDonald K, Hernandez-Boussard T. Electronic health records and quality of care: an observational study modeling impact on mortality, readmissions, and complications. *Medicine (Baltimore).* 2016;95(19):e3332. doi:10.1097/MD.0000000000003332

71. Selvaraj S, Fonarow GC, Sheng S, et al. Association of electronic health record use with quality of care and outcomes in heart failure: an analysis of get with the guidelines-heart failure. *J Am Heart Assoc.* 2018 30;7(7):e008158. doi:10.1161/JAHA.117.008158

72. DesRoches C, Charles D, Furukawa MF, et al. Adoption of electronic health records grows rapidly, but fewer than half of US hospitals had at least a basic system in 2012. *Health Affairs.* 2013;32(8):1478-1485.

73. Lee J, Kuo Y-F, Goodwin JS. The effect of electronic medical record adoption on outcomes in US hospitals. *BMC Health Serv Res.* 2013;13(1):39.

74. Commins J. EHR burdens leave docs burned out, in critical condition. *Health Leaders.* Published September 6, 2016. https://www.healthleadersmedia.com/innovation/ehr-burdens-leave-docs-burned-out-critical-condition?webSyncID=7aa83de1-d989-0483-779d-7e7515957381&sessionGUID=309186d1-2205-2aea-1eae-0191454cdc86&page=0%2C2

75. Young RA, Burge SK, Kumar KA, Wilson JM, Ortiz DF. A time-motion study of primary care physicians' work in the electronic health record era. *Fam Med.* 2018;50(2):91-99. doi:10.22454/FamMed.2018.184803

76. Adler-Milstein J, Zhao W, Willard-Grace R, Knox M, Grumbach K. Electronic health records and burnout: time spent on the electronic health record after hours and message volume associated with exhaustion but not with cynicism among primary care clinicians. *J Am Med Inform Assoc.* 2020;27(4):531-538. doi:10.1093/jamia/ocz220

77. O'Reilly KB. 1 in 3 physicians has been sued; by age 55, 1 in 2 hit with suit. *American Medical Association.* Published January 26, 2018. https://www.ama-assn.org/practice-management/sustainability/1-3-physicians-has-been-sued-age-55-1-2-hit-suit

78. Schaffer AC, Jena AB, Seabury SA, Singh H, Chalasani V, Kachalia A. Rates and characteristics of paid malpractice claims among US physicians by specialty, 1992-2014. *JAMA Intern Med.* 2017;177(5):710-718. doi:10.1001/jamainternmed.2017.0311

79. Studdert DM, Bismark MM, Mello MM, Singh H, Spittal MJ. Prevalence and characteristics of physicians prone to malpractice claims. *N Engl J Med.* 2016;374(4):354-362. doi:10.1056/NEJMsa1506137

80. *MEDPLI.* 2022 Maryland physician's guide to medical malpractice insurance. https://medpli.com/2021-maryland-physicians-guide-to-medical-malpractice-insurance/

81. The Facts About: New York state medical malpractice coverage premiums: 2013-2014 standard medical malpractice premium rates. *Excellus.* Spring 2014. https://truecostofhealthcare.org/wp-content/uploads/2015/02/NewYorkMediMalRates.pdf

82. Eisenberg T. The empirical effects of tort reform. In: Arlen J, ed. *Research Handbook on the Economics of Torts*. 2013. http://papers.ssrn.com/sol3/papers.cfm?abstract_id=2032740

83. DeVito S, Jurs A. An overreaction to a nonexistent problem: empirical analysis of tort reform from the 1980s to 2000s. *Stan J Complex Litig*. 2015;3:62.

84. Mello MM, Frakes MD, Blumenkranz E, Studdert DM. Malpractice liability and health care quality: a review. *JAMA*. 2020;323(4):352-366. doi:10.1001/jama.2019.21411

85. Kachalia A, Kaufmann SR, Boothman R, et al. Liability claims and costs before and after implementation of a medical error disclosure program. *Ann Intern Med*. 2010;153(4):213-221.

86. Mello MM, Kachalia A, Studdert DM. Administrative compensation for medical injuries: lessons from three foreign systems. *The Commonwealth Fund*. Published July 2011. https://www.commonwealthfund.org/publications/issue-briefs/2011/jul/administrative-compensation-medical-injuries-lessons-three

5

Research, Pharmaceuticals, and Medical Devices

Questions as you read through the chapter:

1. How does research funding get distributed? How *should* it be distributed?
2. There are a lot of drugs and devices out there. How do we trust what we use is safe?
3. What is good regulation? What is bad regulation? How do we know?
4. What are good outcomes from collaborations between researchers and industry? What might be bad outcomes? How do we know what kind of collaboration is good or bad? Does industry funding always make a researcher less trustworthy?
5. What kinds of medical innovation should we want to incentivize as a society? How much should we be willing to pay for innovation (in money, in trade-offs, etc)?

Many books about health care and health policy skip over information on research, pharmaceuticals, and medical devices. However, these endeavors form the foundation of health care. In this chapter, you'll gain an overview of these important topics.

Biomedical and Health Research

Medical research is highly variable in multiple dimensions, spanning from scientists with PhDs in a multitude of fields, to physicians and nurses, to statisticians and epidemiologists. The process of scientific discovery is messy, involving a lot of ideas and work that doesn't pan out, and sometimes incredibly slow. It depends on collaboration, competition, mutual learning, and skepticism.

What Are the Types of Research, and How Do They Get Done?

Literally everything can be studied, and so biomedical and health research spans multiple fields and an enormous variety of areas of study. We can think of research as falling into four major categories, shown here with an example of a journal article related to COVID-19. Notice how each example zooms out farther, with the lens expanding from a focus on cells, then to individuals, then to groups, then to society and the environment.

Basic, Bench, or Lab: *Receptor Binding and Complex Structures of Human ACE2 to Spike RBD from Omicron and Delta SARS-CoV-2*, in Cell

Clinical: *Therapeutic Anticoagulation with Heparin in Critically Ill Patients with Covid-19*, in the New England Journal of Medicine

Health Services: *Larger Nursing Home Staff Size Linked to Higher Number of COVID-19 Cases in 2020*, in Health Affairs

Public Health: *Linkages Between Air Pollution and the Health Burden From COVID-19: Methodological Challenges and Opportunities*, in the American Journal of Epidemiology

In terms of clinical research, which is of most interest to us in this chapter, different types of studies represent different ways of asking a research question. These also represent a bit of a hierarchy in terms of how strongly we should accept the conclusions. Although all are necessary in different contexts, the "gold standard" of research is the double-blind randomized controlled trial (RCT). An example of a double-blind RCT experiment would be one in which research patients were randomly assigned to either receive an experimental medication or to receive a sugar pill (placebo), and neither the doctors giving the medication nor the patients themselves know which group is getting which type of pill (ie, both are "blind") (Table 5.1).

Table 5.1 Levels of Research Evidence

Systematic review and meta-analyses	Combines and statistically analyzes data from multiple studies
(*Experimental studies*) Randomized controlled trial	Compares outcomes from a group that receives the treatment to a group that does not
(*Observational studies*) Cohort study, case-control study, cross-sectional study, case reports	Looks either in the past or in the future at what happens to a group of people, or even a single person

Beyond the wide variety in the types of research, there is variety in who does research and where. Each of the articles listed previously may have included the input of academics and scientists, physicians, nurses, epidemiologists, and statisticians. They may have worked at academic institutions, government agencies, private industry, or a private nonprofit.

Who Funds Research?

Research spending rose from $60 billion in 1994[1] to $194 billion in 2018,[2] representing 5% of total spending on health care in the United States. That 5% is mostly funded by private industry research and development (R&D) as well as the federal government, as shown in Figure 5.1.[2]

How Is Funding Distributed?

Nearly $200 billion in funding gets scattered quite widely. Regarding the 22% from the federal government, the National Institutes of Health (NIH)

Where Research and Development (R&D) Funds Come From, 2018

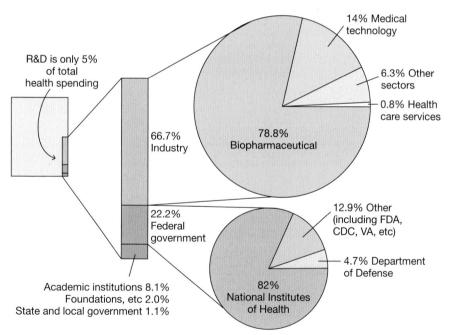

Figure 5.1 CDC, Centers for Disease Control and Prevention; FDA, Food and Drug Administration; VA, Veterans Affairs. (Adapted from Research America. U.S. investments in medical and health research and development 2013-2018. Published Fall 2019. https://www.researchamerica.org/sites/default/files/Publications/InvestmentReport2019_Fnl.pdf)

Table 5.2 National Institutes of Health Funding of Selected Conditions

Topic	2020 funding in millions
Genetics	$10,544
Obesity	$1,145
Colorectal cancer	$319
Malaria	$211
Acute respiratory distress syndrome	$158
Fragile X syndrome	$41
Scleroderma	$24

publishes the estimated distribution of their funding by research topic.[a] Here, we share a short, random list of examples in Table 5.2.

Funding often reflects severity or prevalence of disease. For instance, the NIH distributed at least $4.9 billion for COVID-19 research,[3] and during the first year and a half of the pandemic about 2,500 articles about COVID-19 were published weekly (totaling nearly 200,000 articles).[4]

Funding can also reflect societal biases. For instance, let's compare funding for cystic fibrosis versus sickle cell disease. Even though sickle cell disease affects more people (about 100,000 in the United States, predominantly Black) than does cystic fibrosis (about 30,000 in the United States, predominantly White), cystic fibrosis research is much better funded. Look at research funding for these two diseases, averaged between 2008 and 2017[5] in Table 5.3.

Discrepancies like this are examples of the social determinants of health (SDoH) discussed in Chapter 1. It is also an example of why research funding

Table 5.3 Comparison of Funding Between Cystic Fibrosis and Sickle Cell Disease

	Cystic fibrosis	Sickle cell anemia
Total NIH funding	$84 million	$76 million
NIH funding per affected person	$2,807	$812
Philanthropic spending	$231 million	$9 million
Drug development	6	2

NIH, National Institutes of Health.

---

[a]Which you can find at https://report.nih.gov/funding/categorical-spending#/

can be controversial—and why lobbying—or getting one's "piece of the pie"—represents an enormous effort and priority for many disease-specific organizations. (You're probably familiar with the pink ribbons for breast cancer awareness, but did you know that periwinkle ribbons are for pulmonary hypertension and zebra print are for neuroendocrine tumors?)

Regulation
Making sure research is safe

Unfortunately, there are many examples of how research on people has caused active harm through history.[b] Human subject research is now heavily regulated to protect the privacy, health, and consent of those being studied. Depending on the type of research and how it's funded, research may be regulated by the government, the institution where it's being conducted, or both. Beyond safety, there are mechanisms in place to set a quality standard for what gets published. Anyone who wants to conduct and publish research is going to need to go through these safeguards.

Federal Oversight: Office of Research Integrity (ORI)—This is a branch of the federal Department of Health & Human Services, charged by Congress with maintaining regulatory oversight on research. It regulates all research except that subject to the Food and Drug Administration (FDA).

Local Oversight: Institutional Review Boards (IRBs)—These peer review bodies of medical professionals, often multidisciplinary, are charged with protecting the safety and welfare of human subjects in medical research and clinical trials. IRBs focus primarily on protecting potential research subjects and must approve protocols, consent forms, etc. You'll find these at every institution that conducts medical research, as all research that involves humans (even if only collecting data from their medical records) requires approval from an IRB. IRBs are required to have at least one non-scientist member and at least one member unaffiliated with the research institution.

The Law: Health Insurance Portability and Accountability Act (HIPAA)—If you work in the health professions, you know something about HIPAA, which enacted the first universal code in the United States to protect patient privacy. HIPAA protects patient confidentiality and informed consent, regulating how patients' personal health information can be viewed, stored, and used in both clinical care and research. The federal government keeps a public accounting of privacy breaches affecting 500 or more people.[c]

---

[b]If you ever engage in human subject research, you'll take a short course that reviews this history.
[c]You can look it up here: https://ocrportal.hhs.gov/ocr/breach/breach_report.jsf

Making sure research is high quality: peer review

"Science" is a process of searching for truth by asking questions and studying what happens when you try things. Not all of what comes out of this process is well done. Medical peer review seeks to hold science to a high standard by requiring that knowledgeable colleagues critique the validity of the data, assumptions, and design of research studies before those studies can be published. Articles submitted to scientific journals are judged by (volunteer) researchers whose expertise is in the same field. Each reviewer is given an advance copy of the article and may accept it as is (rare), request revisions (sometimes), or reject the article (often). Reviewers are expected to recuse themselves if they are working on the same project or cannot provide an objective analysis, so that a conflict of interest (COI) will not bias the review.

What Have We Gotten for All This Research?

Researchers estimate that roughly 50% of longevity gains in the past century can be attributed to medical care.[6] The medical research system has built and bolstered that care. David Cutler, a Harvard economist, gives an idea of the value of medical research by focusing on cardiovascular disease, the number one cause of death.[7]

Cutler tells us (a) that research in cardiovascular disease has produced high- and low-tech innovation, and behavioral changes causing health improvements; (b) that such health improvements have increased average life expectancy by 4.5 years; and (c) that the amount of research dollars spent for longevity gain means funding research is a great deal. To quote:

> The average 45 year old spends about $30,000 more currently on cardiovascular disease than he or she did in 1950. But the gains from longer life are much greater. Using common values in the literature, we estimate that the improved health resulting from medical treatment changes is approximately $120,000. The rate of return to medical technology innovation is therefore about 4 to 1. The return to new knowledge is even greater. We estimate that basic knowledge about disease risk has a return of about 30 to 1.[14]

In Figure 5.2, we use the development of the cholesterol-lowering drugs statins as an example of how the expansion of fundamental scientific knowledge connects with and leads to the application of that knowledge to improve health. Scientists learned about cholesterol and the human body for a 100 years, and researchers tried out medical compounds for 25 years, before the first statin medication was approved and sold on the market. Today, researchers continue to learn about the best use of cholesterol-lowering medications as well as other strategies to reduce cardiovascular mortality.

From Bench to Bedside: The Discovery and Development of Statin Drugs

1888
Molecular formula of
cholesterol is established.

1910s
First evidence of connecting cholesterol
with plaques in arteries

1950s
Epidemiologic connection between people who have heart attacks and higher levels of
blood cholesterol. Pathway of cholesterol synthesis in the body is established.

1960s
Search for a drug to block cholesterol synthesis, including the role of HMG-CoA
reductase. Some medications tried but stopped because of side effects.

1970s
Testing compounds that block HMG-CoA reductase (ie, statins)
both in cells and in animals. First testing in humans with compactin,
stopped for side effects. Lovastatin developed by Merck.

1981
First Lovastatin testing.

1984
Large phase III
trials of Lovastatin.

1986
Merck submits a New
Drug Application to the
FDA for Lovastatin.

1987
Lovastatin is the first statin
medication sold on the market.

1990s
More statins come to market, many studies of their effects
are conducted, and guidelines for their use are developed.

2001
Lovastatin goes generic. Statin use increases from 12.5 million
Americans in 2000 to 24 million in 2004.

2016
The last statin goes generic. Almost 30% of adults
over age 40 take a statin, and over $16 billion is
spent on statins annually.

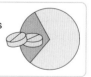

Figure 5.2 FDA, Food and Drug Administration; HMG-CoA, 3-hydroxy-3-
methylglutaryl coenzyme A.

Another salient example of the research contribution to health—on an even more expedited timeline—is the development of COVID-19 messenger ribonucleic acid (mRNA) vaccines. Although mRNA was first discovered in the 1960s, and some testing of its use in therapies began in the 2000s, the world then saw an amazingly quick—and unprecedented—process from sequencing the SARS-CoV-2 genome in January 2020 to large-scale vaccine distribution in January 2021, going from bench to bedside in a year.

Pharmaceuticals and Devices

First, let's talk about pharmaceuticals, which we also interchangeably call medications, drugs, or prescriptions. A pharmaceutical is a chemical substance used to prevent, treat, or cure a disease. In the 1920s, there weren't many drugs beyond aspirin, morphine, and nitroglycerin, whereas today, the 20,000 prescription drugs available in the United States[11] represent a $610 billion industry.[12] Medications are prescribed at two-thirds of office visits, and over half of Americans have taken a prescription in the past month,[13] although, interestingly, one-third of all prescriptions written by providers are never filled by patients.[14]

For the purposes of regulation, pharmaceuticals are usually divided into two groups:

- Small-molecule drugs are chemically synthesized molecules sometimes derived from naturally occurring products. Most prescription drugs available, from Valium to Valsartan to Viagra, are small-molecule drugs.
- Large-molecule drugs, also known as "biologics," are produced by living cells rather than through chemical synthesis. They're larger and more complex than small-molecule pharmaceuticals and, not surprisingly, usually cost a whole lot more. Examples of biologics include insulin, vaccines, and the anticancer drug Avastin.

Both of these groups can be either brand name or generic (called "biosimilar" for the large-molecule drugs). Each individual brand medication is called a New Molecular Entity (NME) by the FDA.

Growth of the Pharmaceutical Industry

Modern medicine is practically synonymous with the development of pharmaceuticals. The history of using medications to treat disease was a slow development over millennia that sped up and then exploded after 1950. In ancient times, healers used herbs to treat disease. The Age of Enlightenment gave rise to modern chemistry, isolating many chemicals that would eventually be used in medications. In 1796, the first precursor to vaccines was used against smallpox. In the 19th century and early 20th century, scientists discovered morphine, aspirin, quinine, adrenaline, phenobarbital, and vitamin C. In the 1920s, insulin was first injected into a human, making it the first biologic. In 1944, penicillin was manufactured on a large scale, completely changing the practice of medicine, only 16 years after it was discovered. By the mid-20th century, researchers and pharmaceutical companies worked together in a fantastic age of discovery and creation, with a boom in medications. The 1990s in particular were an age of "blockbuster" brand name drugs, like Lipitor (atorvastatin) and Prozac (fluoxetine), which drove a huge increase in drug spending (Figure 5.3).

In the past 30 years, we have truly been in the era of Big Pharma. In 2020, the five largest pharmaceutical companies, by revenue,[15-18] are given in Table 5.4.

Intellectual Property

A new drug or device, like any other invention, receives intellectual property (IP) protection from the U.S. government, which is achieved in two ways:

Patents: The purpose of patents is to protect ownership and profit rights for new and innovative inventions. Many aspects of a pharmaceutical or device can be patented, including the molecular structure, method of use, and manufacturing process. For pharmaceuticals, these patents last for 20 years, but most drugs are patented early in development, years before the FDA approves them. The duration of a patent on a new drug can be extended by up to 5 years to compensate for time lost to clinical trials and FDA review. By the time a drug is released to market, it typically has 8 to 14 years of patent protection left. One of the easiest ways for a company to make more money on their drug is to figure out legal ways to extend patents—this is an important strategy for industry with a major impact on patients and society.

Data Exclusivity: For a period of time after a new drug is approved, the safety and efficacy data from its clinical trials cannot be used by generic manufacturers. Small-molecule drugs have data exclusivity for 5 to 7.5 years after approval, whereas biologics have 12 years. Data exclusivity can be extended by filing a supplemental NDA for a new indication (adding 3 years)[d] or a pediatric indication (adding 6 months).

IP protection is meant to ensure that the drug is protected from competition for some time, allowing the manufacturer to recoup its investment.

---

[d]Not available for biologics.

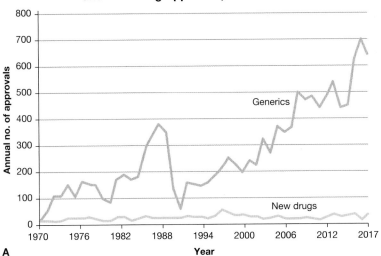

Annual Number of Abbreviated New Drug Applications (ANDAs) and New Drug Approvals, 1970 to 2018

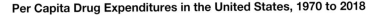

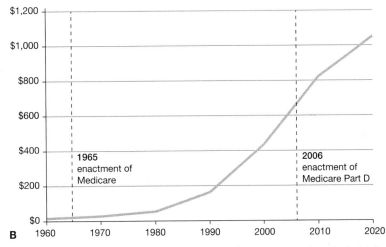

Per Capita Drug Expenditures in the United States, 1970 to 2018

Figure 5.3 "New drugs" include only new molecular entities and exclude biologics, which are not subject to copying via the ANDA pathway. ANDAs include discontinued ANDAs and exclude tentative approvals and approvals with over-the-counter status. Years indicated are calendar years. The surge in ANDA approvals from 1985 to 1988 followed the enactment of the 1984 Hatch-Waxman Act. ANDA approvals prior to the Hatch-Waxman Act occurred pursuant to U.S. Food and Drug Administration regulation. (Data from CMS National Health Expenditures by type of service and source of funds, CY 1960-2020. https://www.cms.gov/Research-Statistics-Data-and-Systems/Statistics-Trends-and-Reports/NationalHealthExpendData/NationalHealthAccountsHistorical; Darrow JJ, Avorn J, Kesselheim AS. FDA approval and regulation of pharmaceuticals, 1983-2018. *JAMA.* 2020;323(2):164-176. doi:10.1001/jama.2019.20288)

Table 5.4 Five Largest Pharmaceutical Companies by Revenue, 2020

Company	Country	Annual revenues	Employees	Top seller[a]
Johnson & Johnson	United States	$82.6 billion	134,500	Stelara
Roche	Switzerland	$58.3 billion	101,465	Avastin
Novartis	Switzerland	$49.9 billion	108,000	Cosentyx
Merck	United States	$48 billion	74,000	Keytruda
AbbVie	United States	$45.8 billion	47,000	Humira

[a]All of these are immune-modulating drugs, used for diseases like cancer and autoimmune disorders.
Sources: Carbajal E. 10 of the largest pharma companies, ranked by 2020 revenue. *Becker's Hospital Review.* Published December 13, 2021. https://www.beckershospitalreview.com/pharmacy/top-10-pharma-companies-by-revenue-in-2020.html; Christel M. 2021 Pharm Exec top 50 companies. *Pharmaceutical Executive.* 2021;41(6). https://www.pharmexec.com/view/2021-pharma-50. Craft. Johnson & Johnson. July 2022. https://craft.co/johnson-johnson. Pistilli M. 10 top pharma companies by revenue. *INN Pharmaceutical Investing News.* Published December 9, 2021. https://investingnews.com/daily/life-science-investing/pharmaceutical-investing/top-pharma-companies-by-revenue/

However, finding the right duration for patent protection and data exclusivity is tricky: longer IP protection keeps low-cost generics off the market, translating to higher prices for patients and payers, whereas a shorter duration would decrease the financial reward for the manufacturer and reduce the incentive to develop new drugs in the future.

Generics and Biosimilars

After the patent for a small-molecule drug has expired, other manufacturers can make their own version of the same molecule; these are dubbed "generic" pharmaceuticals. In 1984, Congress passed the Hatch-Waxman Act, which allowed certain protections for patents of brand name drugs while also incentivizing the development of generic drugs. Generics manufacturers don't get a "recipe" for the brand name drug: they have to reverse-engineer it. Then generic manufacturers must conduct trials to show that their version of the drug is absorbed and distributed in the body in basically the same way as the original drug (that it is "bioequivalent"), but they otherwise have an abbreviated process of approval, without having to repeat all the same clinical trials that the original did. Because the generics manufacturers don't have to invest as much in research and testing, they can sell the generic drug much more cheaply.

In several states, pharmacies can automatically substitute a generic for any bioequivalent prescription unless the provider or patient specifically requests the brand name drug. Today, 89% of all prescriptions are written for generics.[19]

The generic version of a biologic drug is known as a "biosimilar." Biosimilars are much more difficult to create than generics because the manufacturing and purification process for biologics is far more complex than for small-molecule drugs. The Affordable Care Act (ACA) mandated a process for the FDA to approve and regulate biosimilars. The first biosimilar—a medication to increase white blood cells in patients taking toxic chemotherapy drugs—was approved in 2015,[20] and by the end of 2021, there had been at least 30 more biosimilars approved.[21]

What About Medical Devices?

Like pharmaceuticals, medical devices are real-world applications of research. Medical devices can improve health and treatment through:

- Better diagnostics (eg, computed tomography [CT] scans)
- Safer and less invasive procedures (eg, laparoscopic surgery)
- Longer lives (eg, defibrillators)
- Easier lives (eg, full joint replacements)

The number and complexity of available medical devices have increased significantly over the past 25 years. Today, more than $156 billion is spent on medical devices in the United States each year.[22]

How Are the Pharmaceutical and Device Industries Regulated?

The mission of the FDA is to regulate and ensure the safety of goods affecting individual and public health, including food and nutritional supplements, drugs, vaccines and biotechnology, radiation-emitting devices, cosmetics, tobacco products, and veterinary products. The FDA was created in the 1930s; before that, you just had to take on faith that whatever medicine you were purchasing wasn't ineffective "snake oil"—or, worse, poison. A centralized, trustworthy system of ensuring the safety and efficacy of medical treatments is of utmost importance to the entire medical system. Without it, the system could not function. This is what the FDA aims to achieve.

To give an idea of its scope, the FDA regulates about 20% of what U.S. consumers spend money on every year (that's a lot of control over consumer goods!).[11] About 40% of FDA funding goes toward pharmaceuticals and another 10% toward medical devices.[11]

FDA Process for Approving Pharmaceuticals

The path to approval for a new pharmaceutical agent is long and stringent. A manufacturer can apply for a new drug if it is a "new molecular entity" or a previously used molecular entity employed in a new way. The FDA requires several stages of clinical testing before allowing a new drug on the market; each stage adds more data about efficacy and safety. Only about 14% of NMEs end up getting approved and sold—ranging from 3.4% for oncology drugs to 33% for vaccines.[23] Only 53 new drugs passed muster in 2020.[24]

The entire process looks something like this[25]:

■ A pharmaceutical company identifies a promising molecular compound. Testing begins on individual cells, and, if successful, proceeds to testing on live animals. The company can then submit an Investigational New Drug (IND) application to the FDA. The FDA has 30 days to review the IND, and, if approved, trials on human subjects can begin.

■ **Phase I:** The drug is tested on a small group (20-100) of healthy volunteers to make sure it's not immediately toxic and to determine some basic information about how the drug is absorbed and excreted from the body.

■ **Phase II:** The drug is tested on a larger group (30-300) of volunteers, all with the disease the drug targets (eg, familial hypercholesterolemia for lovastatin). This phase continues the experiments from Phase I and starts to assess the drug's safety and efficacy at different doses.

■ **Phase III:** RCTs, usually double-blinded and multicenter, sometimes compared with a competitor, of a large group (300-3,000) of patients with the disease of interest. Half of the patients receive the new drug and half receive a placebo or current gold standard treatment. After a sufficient amount of time, the outcomes of the two groups are compared. Phase III trials are the most expensive and time-consuming part of the approvals process.

■ The manufacturer submits an NDA to the FDA, which contains all information known about the drug, both negative and positive, in all circumstances.

■ The FDA has 10 months to review the application. It may approve it, approve it on condition of Phase IV trials, or reject the application. Once the FDA has approved an NDA, the drug may be sold immediately.

■ **Phase IV:** Postapproval monitoring of a group of patients on the drug to determine side effects and drug interactions. For every drug approved, the manufacturer is required to collect reports of adverse events and drug interactions and submit them in periodic reports to the FDA.[11]

There are several variations and new pathways, though, making the process more complicated but better able to meet needs for drugs with particular priorities (ie, "orphan drugs" for rare diseases, or those warranting expedited review).

If all this feels too complicated, please see the children's book *If You Give a Mouse Metformin*.[e]

FDA Process for Approving Devices

The FDA also regulates the approval and sale of medical devices in the United States. The specifics of the approvals process for each device depend on the level of risk to the patient. The FDA categorizes every device as low (Class I), intermediate (Class II), or high risk (Class III), and the requirements to prove safety and effectiveness vary accordingly. This makes sense—complicated, high-risk devices such as pacemakers ought to go through more testing than simple, low-risk devices such as canes. Low-risk devices simply have to register their devices with the FDA, whereas high-risk devices undergo a process similar to pharmaceuticals.

The FDA also maintains a system for tracking adverse events for products approved and released into the market. Manufacturers are required to report to the FDA any serious device-related adverse events that caused or could have caused serious injury or death. Similar requirements exist for hospitals and other health care facilities. After receiving reports about a specific device, the FDA has a range of options, from further study to mandatory recall. The FDA recalled 57 types of defective devices—like fracture-prone pacemaker wires—in 2021.[26]

You may have heard of Elizabeth Holmes, who in 2021 was convicted of defrauding investors in her biotech company Theranos. Theranos claimed to have developed new blood-testing technology that could accurately analyze results on just a single drop of blood, a much smaller sample than any other technology is capable of. Only, this was a lie: their machines didn't work, and they gave inaccurate results to patients. Holmes and her company had managed to exploit a loophole in FDA regulations that let them fly under the radar of regulatory bodies for a decade, without any oversight of their faulty devices, and the company was first exposed when whistleblowers got the FDA involved for inspections.[27] Theranos is a good example of the importance of regulatory oversight for devices.

How Much Regulation Is the Right Amount?

Many criticize the way the government, specifically the FDA, regulates the pharmaceutical and medical device industries—and the criticisms come from all sides. About 14% of all drugs that make it to FDA clinical trials ultimately win approval and get sold on the market—but is 14% high, low, or just right?[24] If it's low, is it appropriately so (thus protecting us from dangerous or ineffective medications) or inappropriately so (because of a process so difficult that

---

[e]Yes, this is a real book by policy wonk Nikhil Krishnan.

drug costs need to be hiked up for the few that make it through)? Everyone wants safe and effective medications and devices, but it's not obvious how much and what kinds of regulation are necessary to get to that point.

Too much regulation

On the one hand, some think that the FDA has an overly long and costly approvals process, requiring too many hoops to jump through and too much pointless bureaucratic red tape, which ultimately leads to fewer medications available for use. They point to potentially life-saving drugs that people desperately want to try—for instance, to treat cancer or rare diseases—and the "invisible graveyard" of patients who died without access to treatments under investigation.[28] These criticisms were made in 2020, when the FDA shut down early COVID rapid testing devices, and in 2021, when some chastised the FDA for not approving the COVID-19 vaccines earlier. Such critics cite the 9-month delay between emergency use authorization and full approval of the first COVID-19 vaccine, finding this delay to be not only pointless in the face of data indicating safe and effective vaccines, but also life-threatening in that it caused some people to decline to get the vaccine.

Too little regulation

On the other hand, it's extremely important that the FDA conducts its approvals process in a trustworthy and transparent manner. That is, people who wouldn't take the vaccine because they worried about the lack of full FDA approval weren't exactly going to change their minds if they also perceived the FDA to be rushing a slapdash approvals process. In fact, some say the regulation of the FDA is actually too loose. They argue that clinical trials are too short to adequately evaluate for long-term adverse effects. They also argue that important Phase III trial data are kept from public view. Although the FDA began requiring many clinical trials to be publicly posted on clinicaltrials.gov in 2007, investigators have found that a substantial number of researchers fail to comply, without facing consequences from the FDA.[29]

Too much industry influence

In 1992, Congress passed legislation, the Prescription Drug User Fee Act (known by the charming acronym PDUFA), to speed up the FDA drug approvals process. This legislation set specific deadlines for the FDA reviews of new pharmaceuticals. To pay for the extra staff needed to meet these deadlines, PDUFA also mandated a fee system for pharmaceutical companies that submit drugs for FDA review. Although PDUFA did succeed in reducing the amount of time that drugs spend in the approvals process, it also has generated controversy. Fees paid by pharmaceutical companies now account for 65% of the FDA budget for drug review,[11] meaning, essentially, that the FDA is funded by the industry that it regulates. Similar legislation for the medical device industry (called MDUFMA, naturally) was enacted in 2002. At a minimum, this setup creates the appearance that the FDA has a major COI in regard to drug and device regulation.

Problems with a global market

The FDA doesn't just approve medications—it also aims to ensure the ongoing safety of their manufacture. There are thousands and thousands of large pharmaceutical manufacturing plants, and many, particularly for generics, are located outside the United States. The growth of this global industry has been so large that, in 2008, the FDA began opening offices in other countries, such as China and India,[30] and by 2021, nearly half of all drugs and devices were manufactured outside the United States.[11] But the FDA has no legal authority in other countries, limiting the effectiveness of inspections and oversight. Further, even if drugs are manufactured in American plants, their ingredients might not be: 78% of all active pharmaceutical ingredients are manufactured outside the United States.[11] The FDA focuses on ensuring a good manufacturing process rather than testing all products—because it simply can't. Even so, the oversight necessary to evaluate materials and drugs on a global market strains the staffing, budget, and authority of the FDA. The discovery of impurities led to the recall of 195 drugs from 2017 to 2019[31]—many of these common medications for things like heartburn and hypertension.

Another shocking example is detailed in the book *Bottle of Lies* by Katherine Eban,[32] which tells of the Indian generics manufacturer Ranbaxy, the first overseas manufacturer to sell generic drugs in the United States. In 2005, a whistleblower had alerted the FDA to lack of quality assurance, impurities, and outright fraud at Ranbaxy manufacturing plants. The FDA was under a lot of pressure to allow Ranbaxy to sell a generic alternative to Pfizer's brand name atorvastatin ("Lipitor") after it went off-patent in 2011, because a generic to this blockbuster cholesterol-lowering medication would save the government quite a bit of money. After a very long investigation and legal battle, Ranbaxy USA agreed to pay $500 million to the FDA in 2013—while continuing to sell many of the medications called into question (in fact, Ranbaxy held exclusive rights to sell generics for the first 6 months after Lipitor's patent expired). Eban's book cites continued concerns not just about Ranbaxy, but about the FDA's generally limited ability to curtail bad manufacturing process and fraud in a global market.

Paying for Prescription Drugs

Most insurance covers prescription drugs, though notably in Medicare it's optional to purchase the Part D prescription drug benefit. Prescription coverage is similar in many ways to other aspects of insurance as discussed in Chapter 2, including cost-sharing, but it differs in some key ways. Let's go through these in an example: say you develop asthma, and your doctor prescribes you a brand name asthma inhaler called Advair. The doctor doesn't think anything of it—Advair is a common medication that's been available since 2000—and neither do you. Sticker shock ensues when the pharmacy tells you that a single Advair inhaler is priced at $470,[f] even though you have insurance. Why did this happen?

The flow of money for prescription drugs is (surprise, surprise!) quite complex. Nearly all insurance types cover prescription medications. Legally, insurers are often required to cover all prescription options for certain conditions—and Medicaid is required to cover all FDA-approved medications, period—but generally private insurers can negotiate prices with manufacturers and decline to cover some medications altogether. The list of covered medications is called a formulary,[g] which probably includes Advair but might not. (Hospitals also use formularies for inpatients—so a hospital might *only* give a generic inhaler, even if you take Advair at home.)

All of this is made more complicated by Pharmacy Benefits Managers (PBMs). PBMs act as middlemen, typically contracting with a large number of insurers to consolidate negotiating power against manufacturers, ostensibly to reduce drug costs for the insurance payers (see Chapter 3 for more about PBMs). Interestingly, Medicare, despite being the nation's largest insurer, has historically missed out on this negotiating power even though it is such a large insurer, because it contracted out its Part D prescription drug benefit to many private plans and was barred from establishing a national formulary or negotiating prices in a centralized manner.[h,33]

Beyond negotiating a formulary, payers and PBMs have other methods to steer patients toward cheaper drugs. These methods, called "drug utilization management," work by increasing the barriers to more expensive drugs.

1. Step therapy: requiring patients to have tried another (cheaper to the payer) drug first

---

[f]According to GoodRx, this is the average retail price of Advair. A generic of Advair (fluticasone-salmeterol) was approved in 2019, but this will still run you about $350, according to GoodRx.
[g]Some specialty drugs—frequently but not always biologics—are not picked up at pharmacies but require an infusion at a health care facility. Because of this, some plans (including Medicare) cover these medications as outpatient care rather than as a prescription drug benefit.
[h]Please see "A Note on the Inflation Reduction Act" at the beginning of this book.

2. Prior authorization: requiring paperwork from clinicians to demonstrate that a patient really needs the more expensive drug ("justify" the use)

3. Higher cost-sharing from patients

Then things get even more complicated because of rebates. Rebates are supposed to get payers (or sometimes patients) money back for spending on expensive drugs. Manufacturers can offer rebates to PBMs, to patients themselves, and, under a law called 340B Drug Discounting Program, *must* offer discounts to certain hospitals and clinics, usually in the safety net.

It sounds good to have strategies to reduce drug spending. But do these methods actually reduce health care costs overall? Drug utilization management creates a huge administrative burden, with costs both to individual physician's offices (each prior authorization "costs" the office ~$6-15 to deal with[34]) as well as spread across payers, patients, and PBMs themselves (estimated at a total of $93.3 billion[35]). Further, discounts and rebates can lower prices in particular instances—being literally life-saving for patients—without lowering the overall *system* of high spending. In fact, one study suggests that rebates for brand drugs actually raise demand and shift price negotiations for an overall *increase* in those drugs' prices by 30%.[36] (And, for their part, PBMs have been criticized for keeping too much of the rebate for themselves.[37])

A few companies cut through all the chaos in Figure 5.4. (Find Figure 5.4 confusing? Yup, that's because the payment system is chaos!) One is Walmart, with its well-known $4 list.[i] Walmart purchases over 100 generic medications from wholesalers and then sells them directly to consumers (without billing insurance). Another is Civica Rx, a not-for-profit generics manufacturer founded in 2018. Civica Rx makes and sells drugs that have a shortage, like antibiotics and anesthetics, primarily doing business with hospitals. Another well-known company, GoodRx, cuts insurance out of the equation but continues to rely on the complicated relationship between pharmacies and PBMs to offer discounted rates directly to consumers.[38] More recently, both Amazon and Cost Plus[39] are attempting to do the same. All of these can be lifelines for patients without insurance or with high copays, but again they do not fix the underlying system of high prices.[40]

Back to our asthma inhaler example. Your insurance won't pay for Advair but will cover a similar inhaler in the same medication class, called Symbicort. This is because the payer's PBM negotiated a better rate with AstraZeneca, which makes Symbicort, than with GlaxoSmithKline, which makes Advair. You might still be able to get Advair if your clinician submits a prior authorization. You might even be able to find a coupon or payment assistance program, such as from GoodRx or from GlaxoSmithKline itself, that brings the cost of

---

[i]Although they actually charge up to $15.

Conceptual Model of the Flow of Products, Services, and Funds for Nonspecialty Drugs Covered Under Private Insurance and Purchased in a Retail Setting

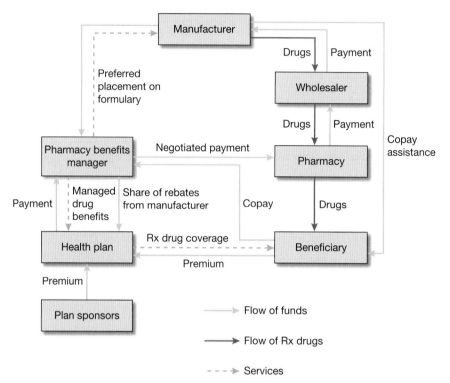

Figure 5.4 Adapted from Sood N, Shih T, Nuys KV, Goldman D. Flow of money through the pharmaceutical distribution system. *USC Schaeffer.* Published June 6, 2017. https://healthpolicy.usc.edu/research/flow-of-money-through-the-pharmaceutical-distribution-system/

the Advair inhaler down. But probably you don't care enough about Advair to go through all that, so your doctor prescribes Symbicort instead. Now, you'll just pay your copay, which for Symbicort is an average of approximately $32 per month.[41] But, unfortunately, you might go through this process again next year, when your payer's PBM renegotiates with manufacturers and changes its formulary. Now they want you to take Advair instead of Symbicort.

For some, that sticker shock never does wear off. Estimates differ, but around 16% of adults don't fill their prescriptions because of cost.[42] For more reading on this topic, please see Section "Pharmacies" in Chapter 1, Section "Growth of Middlemen: Spotlight on PBMs" in Chapter 3, Section "Drug Pricing Controversies" in this chapter, and Section "Aduhelm controversy" in Chapter 6.

Issues

We will now turn to a few controversies plaguing the world of research and industry—and we'll end with a long discussion of drug pricing, itself a confusing area of research, opinion, and failed policy.

Research Validity Concerns

Scientific research is susceptible to many problems, including:

- Researchers may frame their questions in a way that points to predetermined conclusions.
- They may choose a poorly representative population sample.
- They may make a mistake in data analysis.
- Intentional fraud may skirt past peer review, which is not designed to detect it.[j]
- A journal may publish or reject articles for reasons other than the validity of the science.
- The media may report conclusions that aren't truly demonstrated by the study.
- The study may be invalidated later but never retracted in the eyes of other researchers and the public.[k]

Further, science barrels forward, and studies may quickly go out of date as new methods and materials are introduced. No matter how exacting and hard-working scientists may be, there's no perfect research study. Thus, a growing number of scientists—the most famous of whom is John Ioannadis—have begun to study not only biomedical questions, but also the research world itself and how it's affected by the problems listed. Some of their findings are startling:

- Many studies are refuted at a later date. Of the 49 most influential studies during a 13-year period, 45 of them found an intervention to be effective. Of those 45, 32% have subsequently been shown to be wrong or exaggerated.[43,44]
- Researchers are more likely to submit, and journals are more likely to publish, experiments with positive results,[45,46] termed "publication bias." Five identical experiments may only produce the desired result once; but if that

---

[j]One woman, Elisabeth Bik, has gained some fame by dedicating herself to finding fraud in journal images. https://www.nature.com/articles/d41586-020-01363-z

[k]Although the site Retraction Watch monitors just this with a database of retracted papers, mostly in the life sciences. https://retractionwatch.com/

one trial is the only one submitted and published, the general public would have the false impression that 100% of the experiments were successful.[1]

■ COI may arise. New medical and pharmaceutical products are subject to multiple trials to prove efficacy and safety. Yet many of these studies are funded by the very same company that produces the product. Not surprisingly, trials funded by a private company are more likely—4 times as much, in one major study[47]—to have results that benefit the sponsoring company than are trials funded by others.

■ The research system lacks a consistent way to retract published research later determined to be invalid. Researchers often continue to cite the results of invalid papers for many years after they have been retracted; even more surprising, many papers found to be fraudulent are never retracted at all.[48]

In other words, as Mark Twain may or may not have said, "There are three kinds of lies: lies, damned lies, and statistics." Which isn't to say that research evidence isn't true, but rather that published results data or research conclusion isn't unquestionable proof, given that the way that result was developed and interpreted might be faulty.

Nothing could underscore this point—and the downstream effects of flawed or fraudulent research—more than the story of Andrew Wakefield.[49] In 1998, Wakefield and colleagues published a case series in the journal *Lancet* suggesting a link between the measles, mumps, and rubella vaccine and autism. Subsequent research found no link, and it turned out Wakefield had hidden COI as well as misrepresented the study design; the paper was fully retracted by *Lancet* 2010. A year later, investigations found that Wakefield had committed deliberate fraud and was completely discredited in the scientific community. But we all know that his fraudulent claims lived on, fueling a growing skepticism about vaccines that ended up, more than 20 years after Wakefield's study was published, convincing millions of Americans not to get vaccinated against COVID-19. Understanding research design and statistics is difficult, and even clinicians might not be well versed in it, much less the general public, but it is extremely important to health care that research evidence be valid and trustworthy.

Conflict of Interest (COI)

The worlds of academics and industry intersect, interact, and overlap. Any time you have an intermingling of groups with diverse motivations—mixed with billions of dollars—COIs are bound to arise. Academic researchers investigating a

---

[1]To counteract publication bias, the NIH has created a publicly available trial registry at www.Clinical Trials.gov. There, researchers can prospectively catalog their trials and report basic results after completion, even if the research isn't published in a journal. The FDA and several consortiums of medical journals now require many trials to be registered at ClinicalTrials.gov.

new drug or device are often funded by the very same company that makes and sells the said product. Pharmaceutical and device companies pay health care providers and researchers to participate in speakers' bureaus and conferences and to consult about new products. They fund conferences and educational groups. About 70,000 pharmaceutical sales representatives are employed to visit physicians' offices to market drugs and distribute free samples.[50]

Publicity about COI in medicine led to the Physician Payments Sunshine Act, a federal law passed in 2010. This act requires companies to report any gift or payment to a physician that is worth $10 or more. The federal government then posts the records of these payments[65] online for public review at the Centers for Medicare & Medicaid Services (CMS) Open Payments website.[m] Physicians began restricting visits from pharma sales reps, with fewer than half allowing access by 2017.[51] Yet, industry connections and payments to physicians haven't gone away. In a high-profile example, in 2018, journalists reported on the millions that prominent oncology researcher Jose Baselga made from the pharmaceutical and device industry, leading to his resignation as chief medical officer of cancer center Memorial Sloan Kettering.[52] Further, a small but significant minority of prescribing physicians receive payments related to some of the medications they prescribe. Notably, over 20% of providers who prescribed oxycontin had a promotional interaction of some sort with manufacturer Purdue Pharmaceuticals[53] (see Section "Opioid Epidemic" in Chapter 6).

Let's look at an example of how COI can be subtle and unclear. In Chapter 6, we talk about policy outlawing surprise billing, which are large bills sent to patients by out-of-network physicians, occurring when physicians (and groups employing them, like private equity) couldn't agree on rates. Much of this policy was informed by 2016 research showing the billing markup by out-of-network physicians/groups. Although this research was performed by independent academics at Yale, it was funded by UnitedHealthCare—a group obviously interested in making physician groups rather than insurance companies out to be the bad guys, and in using negative coverage to improve their standing in negotiations—which journalists claim influenced elements of the study design.[54] Some might think that banning surprise billing is a good outcome regardless of who funded the study, and that the issue is obviously larger and more important than a single study, even if the study was flawed. Others (like those opposing the No Surprises law) might claim that COI led to unfair study results and unfair media coverage resulting in a law that favors insurance companies over physicians in negotiations. In the big picture, one might feel that an individual case like this one is not a big deal in terms of COI, but that the overall system of industry funding of research likely leads to more frequently compromised results.

---

[m]You can look up your own clinician at https://openpaymentsdata.cms.gov/

Although expensive dinners with drug reps may seem like an obvious COI to be outlawed, potential problems because of professional interactions involving research among physicians, researchers, professors, and industry are harder to tease out. Many feel there's a lack of evidence to demonstrate that relationships between physicians, researchers, and industry actually lead to worse health outcomes for patients.

Drug Pricing Controversies

Why do drugs cost so much in the United States, and what can we do about it? These are simple questions with only complicated, controversial, and partial answers. Let's walk through some of the facts and arguments.

Drugs cost a lot, and the total amount spent on them is increasing faster than inflation

Nationwide, inflation-adjusted prescription drug spending increased nearly 8-fold from 1980 to 2018, increasing from $140 to $1,073 per capita in that time.[55] For Medicare patients, annual per capita prescription drug spending reached $2,700 by 2018.[55] Rising costs are a problem for treatments of common chronic conditions, such as insulin for diabetes, and inhalers for asthma—but they are particularly notable for life-saving cancer treatments and biologic immunotherapies. Notice the *logarithmic* scale in Figure 5.5. Note Table 5.5 as well, which lists several brand name drugs that account for a significant portion of drug spending—look at both the current price as well as the amount of increase since they came to market.

R&D costs are also high

There are different estimates of what it costs to bring a single drug to market, ranging from $110 million (in 2001 dollars, from watchdog group Public Citizen)[56] to $928 million (in 2020 dollars, accounting for failed trials[57]) to $2.8 billion (in 2013 dollars, from Tufts University using industry numbers).[58] Costs include designing, testing, and manufacturing, but the majority of R&D costs go toward funding large Phase III clinical trials required by the FDA. The likelihood that a drug undergoing clinical testing will end up being approved and sold is estimated at 12%.[59] That's a lot of costs having to be recouped from the few drugs that do end up being sold.

An important aside here is that drug companies also spend a lot on marketing. Companies market to prescribers—but they also market directly to consumers (something only the United States and New Zealand allow). Annual total spending by drug companies to market prescription drugs is $29.6 billion.[60] One study looking at ten major pharmaceutical companies found that seven of them spent more on marketing each year than they did on R&D.[61]

Price at Time of FDA Approval in 2014 Dollars

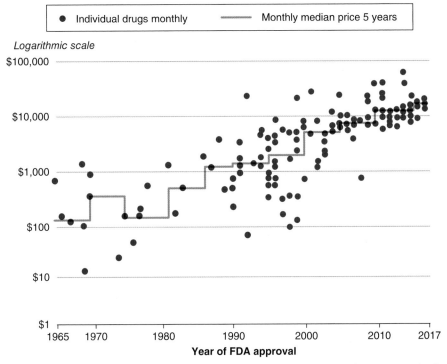

Figure 5.5 FDA, Food and Drug Administration. Source: Peter B. Bach, MD, Memorial Sloan Kettering Cancer Center. (Adapted from Belluz J. The Nobel Prize is a reminder of the outrageous cost of curing cancer. *Vox.* Updated October 2, 2018. https://www.vox.com/science-and-health/2018/10/1/17923720/immunotherapy-cancer-cost)

High drug costs have a negative impact on individuals as well as on society

About 25% of people taking prescription medications say they have trouble affording them.[62] Some people never even get past the sticker shock to purchase the medication at all. Hospitals, too, feel the brunt of high drug costs, with average drug spending per admission increasing by nearly 20% from 2015 to 2017.[63] The burden of this spending falls disproportionately on those with multiple and serious medication conditions as well as high deductibles—but it affects us all, through taxes and offset income.

We could save a lot of money by reducing drug spending

Many options exist to reduce drug spending, but most only do so in dribs and drabs. One notable strategy is by increasing generic rather than brand prescriptions. If a single drug is pricey enough or common enough, a switch to generic can have a major impact. Consider the cholesterol-lowering statins, the

Table 5.5 Price Increases and Revenue, Select Drugs, 2021

Drug	Price (2021)	No. of price increases	Price increase since launch	2019 U.S. net revenue
Humalog (*type of insulin, made by Eli Lilly*)	$274.70/vial	30+	1,219%	$1.67 billion
Lyrica (*treats neuropathy, etc, made by Pfizer*)	$1,200/yr	20+	420%	$2.01 billion
Humira (*immunosuppressant for inflammatory disorders, made by AbbVie*)	$71,600/yr	25+	471%	$14.9 billion
Copaxone (*treats multiple sclerosis, made by Teva*)	$85,400/yr	25+	825%	$950 million
Gleevec (*treats leukemia, made by Novartis*)	$123,000/yr	20+	395%	$330 million

Source: Adapted from Oversight. Drug pricing investigation. majority staff report. Committee on Oversight and Reform U.S. House of Representatives. Published December 2021. https://oversight.house .gov/sites/democrats.oversight.house.gov/files/DRUG%20PRICING%20REPORT%20WITH%20 APPENDIX%20v3.pdf

most popular of which went generic in 2011. Researchers found that Medicare spending on statins decreased by $3 billion from 2014 to 2018 even though more people used them, all just from shifting from brand names to generics. They estimated that we could have saved another $2.1 billion during that time by using generic statins exclusively.[64] However, switching to generics is not a comprehensive solution because (a) many drugs do not have a generic option, and (b) even generics' prices tend to go up when there is limited competition.

But the most effective mechanisms to systematically reduce drug spending are controversial

Drug spending could be substantially reduced by leveraging the federal government's power to:

A. Limit what drugs are covered.
B. Negotiate drug prices on a large scale.

There are both international and domestic precedents for both of these strategies. Most U.S. insurance companies do some form of (A), through drug formularies and prior authorizations; however, these are unpopular and may reflect business deals more than the true cost-effectiveness of medications. Countries like England employ (A) on a national scale based explicitly on

Average Prices Paid by the VA and Medicare for Selected Drugs, 2017

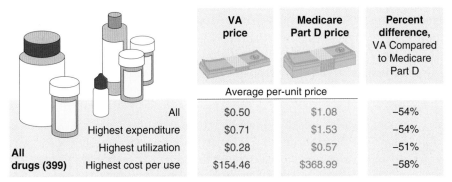

		VA price	Medicare Part D price	Percent difference, VA Compared to Medicare Part D
		Average per-unit price		
	All	$0.50	$1.08	−54%
	Highest expenditure	$0.71	$1.53	−54%
All	Highest utilization	$0.28	$0.57	−51%
drugs (399)	Highest cost per use	$154.46	$368.99	−58%

Figure 5.6   Prices are per-unit, net prices. (Adapted from U.S. Government Accountability Office. Prescription drugs: Department of Veterans Affairs paid about half as much as Medicare part D for selected drugs in 2017. Released January 14, 2021. https://www.gao.gov/products/gao-21-111)

cost-effectiveness, but there is a strong cultural norm against such a practice in the United States. For instance, the ACA created a new research agency to evaluate clinical efficacy of different treatments—called Patient-Centered Outcomes Research Institute (PCORI)—but strictly limited PCORI in how it can evaluate cost-effectiveness.[65]

As for (B), negotiating prices is again the norm. European countries negotiate with drug companies, and they pay a lot less than the United States for the same drugs. And, actually, inside the United States, private payers—as well as the Veterans Affairs (VA)—do the same. The United States could save a lot of money by negotiating on a large scale, like England or the VA does, as shown in Figure 5.6. Yet Medicare, the nation's largest insurer and also a major source of federal spending, has historically been prohibited by law from negotiating drug prices, though this will change beginning in 2023. (See "A Note on the Inflation Reduction Act" at the beginning of this book.)[n]

Why is Medicare negotiating drug prices so controversial?

If you paid attention to the news the past few years, you know that Congress considered, initially rejected, and then ultimately approved a proposal to allow Medicare to negotiate drug prices. (See "A Note on the Inflation Reduction Act" at the beginning of this book.) Why is this issue so controversial? Because the general belief has been that drug creation (ie, innovation) involves such high up-front costs in R&D that the only reason drug companies

---

[n]That is, the individual insurers that Medicare contracts with for Part D may handle their own, small-scale, negotiations, but Medicare cannot centralize those negotiations.

will make the investment is for the promise of high profits. Some argue that European countries who negotiate drug prices are benefiting from the fact that the United States doesn't—that is, Europe is getting a free ride on innovation—and many fear that negotiating prices, by lowering profits, would come at the cost of decreasing future innovation in drug creation.

The debate over whether or not this is true is long-standing, and understanding it is key. Let's frame how to think through the major points and evidence.

We can break the debate down to several questions. So, first, how much innovation is truly innovative? Critics say that the pharmaceutical industry is less innovative than we think. One example is cost-ineffective drugs, such as new cancer drugs that are wildly expensive despite studies showing little if any benefit over older, cheaper therapies. Another example is "me too" drugs, defined as slight variations on an old drug that don't provide any additional clinical benefit—you could also call these copy-cat drugs. Critics ask, do we as a society really need six types of proton pump inhibitors to treat heartburn, or seven forms of statins to lower cholesterol? One expert estimates that only 14% of the 483 new drugs approved between 1998 and 2003 were "new compounds considered likely to be improvements over older drugs."[66,67] Is such redundancy really "innovation"? Yet drug industry defenders say "yes," noting that the statins found to be most effective at preventing heart attacks—atorvastatin and rosuvastatin—were the fourth and fifth statins approved by the FDA.[68]

Second, how much of private sector innovation relies on public investment? A number of laws favor private profits, including a 1980 law called Bayh-Dole, which allows drug companies to patent drugs that were developed using research done at the publicly funded NIH, or at academic institutions but funded by NIH grants. Some claim that, given Bayh-Dole and similar policies, taxpayers "pay twice" for drugs: first by funding basic science research, and second for the full price of the drugs created based on that research. Studies have tried to tease out how much innovation is due to the private sector versus the public sector. Results indicate that about 40% of private sector R&D projects used findings from NIH-funded research, though only 10% to 15% were based solely on that research. Nearly all FDA-approved drugs are linked to government-funded research, though the public sector did enough work such that they would be able to secure a patent themselves in only 20% of "important" drugs. As one expert writes, "One can squarely reject the argument that the public sector role or the private sector roles are zero; indeed both seem to be qualitatively large, important, and complementary."[69]

Third, how much of drug prices actually reflects private industry R&D investment and is necessary for "innovation"? Our evidence here is limited by the secrecy around industry data on both R&D costs as well as pricing; some independent groups have suggested that the true costs of drug creation are lower than the industry numbers, whereas others have agreed with them. Regardless of what R&D cost numbers you believe, the focus on innovation and R&D costs may miss a huge reason why drug prices are high, which is that businesses set prices as high as they can, as with any other market. There have been a few high-profile cases in which drug companies hiked prices on a medication, such as EpiPen, a device that auto-injects the (cheap, old) drug epinephrine into someone having a severe allergic reaction. EpiPen was first approved in the 1980s, and it was priced at approximately $90 when the manufacturing rights were purchased by the drug company Mylan 20 years later. Then, in 2016, Mylan set off a firestorm (and some lawsuits) when they raised the price to approximately $600.[70]

Egregious cases like this get a lot of attention, but the fact is that all drug companies expend a *lot* of energy in finding loopholes to expand patents, extend brand name exclusivity, and reduce competition—all increasing their revenue by keeping prices high. For instance, insulin prices have risen over 1,000% in the past decade (much higher than the 62% rise in inflation),[71] and a 2021 Congressional investigation found that drug companies engaged in anticompetitive, monopoly tactics to raise these prices; see Figure 5.7 for an example of lock-step increases of prices between the two competitors that capture the market.[72]

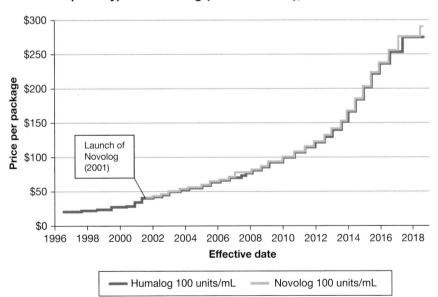

Comparison of Rapid-Acting Insulin Price Increases—Humalog (Eli Lilly) and Novolog (Novo Nordisk), 1996-2018

Figure 5.7 Adapted from Oversight. Drug pricing investigation. majority staff report. Committee on Oversight and Reform U.S. House of Representatives. Published December 2021. https://oversight.house.gov/sites/democrats.oversight.house.gov/files/DRUG%20PRICING%20REPORT%20WITH%20APPENDIX%20v3.pdf

Insulin: an example and imaginary dialogue

Insulin pricing ties together a lot of these issues. Insulin was manufactured in 1922, turning type 1 diabetes mellitus from a universally fatal disease into a chronic one. Famously, the inventors patented it for only $1, believing that medical ethics should prevent the profiting off of a life-saving medication. Fast forward a century: we now have about seven types of insulin and insulin analogs, and the annual cost of insulin for a Medicare patient with diabetes is approximately $5,600.[73]

Person A might say that not only is $5,600 more than any person can be reasonably expected to spend (the uninsured are hit with the full cost), but further that this price increase cannot possibly be justified by R&D "innovation." After all, look at the rise in price for Humalog and Novolog insulin in Figure 5.7. Isn't it galling to pay so much for medications whose invention was publicly funded nearly a century ago?

Yet Person B might counter that, actually, Humalog and Novolog weren't created in the 1920s, and instead are insulin analogs created in the 1990s. Older insulins (called "NPH" and "regular") are still on the market for as little as $25/vial,[o] and there's nothing stopping patients and doctors from using these instead. In fact, the widespread use of the newer, high-priced insulin analogs probably reflects the fact that these are both easier to use and also less likely to cause dangerous low blood sugar—thus reflecting a true innovation worth paying extra for.

Fine, Person A might reply, maybe Humalog is an improvement worth paying for—but how much more? And besides, Humalog sure didn't become *more* innovative after it was approved in 1996, so why did the price increase 10-fold in 20 years? Isn't this an example of how prices don't necessarily reflect R&D costs?

Hold up, says Person C. This whole argument about innovation misses the point. Someone with insulin-dependent diabetes will die without insulin. We as a society have a responsibility to ensure that people don't die just because they cannot afford easily available treatments, as happened to Alec Raeshawn Smith in Minnesota.[74]

It is you who is missing the point, says Person D. If we don't adequately incentivize pharmaceutical companies, then they won't invest in innovative R&D, and we won't get future potential life-saving treatments. The Europeans may find it palatable to cut their own costs when we are footing the bill of innovation. We as a society have a responsibility to our children and grandchildren to ensure more drugs get created.

But, says Person E, if you think that we are purchasing "X" amount of innovation with "Y" current prices, then why not pay even more than we pay

---

[o]Some insulin is even available for purchase without a prescription.

now? Why not double our drug spending to get double the innovation? It just doesn't work that way: there's not a 1:1 correlation between prices and innovation. Plus, it's not like people who want Medicare to negotiate drug prices think they should gouge the drug companies and make them go broke. They just think drug companies shouldn't be able to name whatever price they want.

Person F pokes his head through the door. "Can you guys be quiet? I'm trying to sleep."

So what do we do?

There is, at least, some hope on the insulin front: Civica Rx, the not-for-profit generic manufacturer, plans to start selling generic insulin in 2024 for $30 per vial, with plans to take on more medications in the future.[75] And the Inflation Reduction Act, passed in 2022, will allow Medicare to negotiate some drug prices. But is that enough to fix an entire system? Negotiating drug prices is one obvious strategy, but there are more,[76] none of which is perfect, comprehensive, or universally popular. Ultimately, what you think about these issues probably has a lot to do with your opinions about capitalism and the role of government in ensuring public goods. We have our opinions, but we'll let you make up your own mind.

References

1. Moses H, Matheson DHM, Cairns-Smith S, George BP, Palisch C, Dorsey ER. The anatomy of medical research: US and international comparisons. *JAMA*. 2015;313(2):174-189. doi:10.1001/jama.2014.15939

2. Research America. U.S. investments in medical and health research and development 2013-2018. Published Fall 2019. https://www.researchamerica.org/sites/default/files/Publications/InvestmentReport2019_Fnl.pdf

3. National Institutes of Health. COVID-19 funded research projects. Accessed December 12, 2021. https://covid19.nih.gov/funding

4. LitCovid. A literature hub for tracking up-to-date scientific information about the 2019 novel Coronavirus. Published July 2022. https://www.ncbi.nlm.nih.gov/research/coronavirus/

5. Farooq F, Mogayzel PJ, Lanzkron S, Haywood C, Strouse JJ. Comparison of US federal and foundation funding of research for sickle cell disease and cystic fibrosis and factors associated with research productivity. *JAMA Netw Open*. 2020;3(3):e201737. doi:10.1001/jamanetworkopen.2020.1737

6. Cutler D, Rosen A, Vijan S. The value of medical spending in the United States, 1960-2000. *N Engl J Med*. 2006(355):920-927.

7. Cutler D, Kadiyala S. The return to biomedical research: treatment and behavioral effects. Accessed March 30, 2022. citeseerx.ist.psu.edu/viewdoc/download?doi=10.1.1.200.7197&rep=rep1&type=pdf

8. Endo A. A historical perspective on the discovery of statins. *Proc Jpn Acad Ser B Phys Biol Sci*. 2010;86(5):484-493. doi:10.2183/pjab.86.484

9. Mann D, Reynolds K, Smith D, Muntner P. Trends in statin use and low-density lipoprotein cholesterol levels among US adults: impact of the 2001 National Cholesterol Education Program guidelines. *Ann Pharmacother.* 2008;42(9):1208-1215. doi:10.1345/aph.1L181. https://pubmed.ncbi.nlm.nih.gov/18648016/

10. Lin S, Baumann K, Zhou C, Zhou W, Cuellar AE, Xue H. Trends in use and expenditures for brand-name statins after introduction of generic statins in the US, 2002-2018. *JAMA Netw Open.* 2021;4(11):e2135371. doi:10.1001/jamanetworkopen.2021.35371. https://jamanetwork.com/journals/jamanetworkopen/fullarticle/2786415

11. U.S. Food & Drug Administration. Fact Sheet: FDA at a glance. Accessed July 2022. https://www.fda.gov/about-fda/fda-basics/fact-sheet-fda-glance

12. CNBC. Health and Science. US prescription drug spending as high as $610 billion by 2021: report. Published May 4, 2017. https://www.cnbc.com/2017/05/04/us-prescription-drug-spending-as-high-as-610-billion-by-2021-report.html

13. Centers for Disease Control and Prevention. National Center for Health Statistics. Therapeutic drug use. Accessed July 2022. https://www.cdc.gov/nchs/fastats/drug-use-therapeutic.htm

14. Tamblyn R, Eguale T, Huang A, Winslade N, Doran P. The incidence and determinants of primary nonadherence with prescribed medication in primary care: a cohort study. *Ann Intern Med.* 2014;160(7):441-450.

15. Carbajal E. 10 of the largest pharma companies, ranked by 2020 revenue. *Becker's Hospital Review.* Published December 13, 2021. https://www.beckershospitalreview.com/pharmacy/top-10-pharma-companies-by-revenue-in-2020.html.

16. Christel M. 2021 Pharm Exec top 50 companies. *Pharmaceutical Executive.* 2021;41(6). https://www.pharmexec.com/view/2021-pharma-50.

17. Craft. Johnson & Johnson. July 2022. https://craft.co/johnson-johnson.

18. Pistilli M. 10 top pharma companies by revenue. *INN Pharmaceutical Investing News.* Published December 9, 2021. https://investingnews.com/daily/life-science-investing/pharmaceutical-investing/top-pharma-companies-by-revenue/

19. The generic drug supply chain. *Association of Accessible Medicines.* Accessed July 2022. https://accessiblemeds.org/resources/blog/generic-drug-supply-chain

20. James D. First biosimilar approved in United States. *Pharmacy Times.* Published March 6, 2015. https://www.drugs.com/medical-answers/many-biosimilars-approved-united-states-3463281/

21. Wikipedia. Technically taken from Wikipedia. Cites FDA press releases for each. July 2022.

22. Select USA/SUSA MedTech Industry Associations. Medical Technology Industry. Industry Associations. July 2022. https://www.trade.gov/susa-medtech-industry-associations

23. Wong CH, Siah KW, Lo AW. Estimation of clinical trial success rates and related parameters [published correction appears in *Biostatistics.* 2019 Apr 1;20(2):366]. *Biostatistics.* 2019;20(2):273-286. doi:10.1093/biostatistics/kxx069

24. Mullard A. 2020 FDA drug approvals. *News & Analysis.* https://media.nature.com/original/magazine-assets/d41573-021-00002-0/d41573-021-00002-0.pdf

25. U.S. Food & Drug Administration. The FDA's drug review process: ensuring drugs are safe and effective. Updated November 2017. https://www.fda.gov/drugs/information-consumers-and-patients-drugs/fdas-drug-review-process-ensuring-drugs-are-safe-and-effective

26. U.S. Food & Drug Administration. 2021 Medical device recalls. Updated November 2021. https://www.fda.gov/medical-devices/medical-device-recalls/2021-medical-device-recalls

27. Carreyrou J. *Bad Blood.* Picador; 2019.

28. Tabarrok A. Is the FDA too conservative or too aggressive? *Marginal Revolution*. Economics, Medicine, Science. Published August 26, 2015. https://marginalrevolution .com/marginalrevolution/2015/08/is-the-fda-too-conservative-or-too-aggressive.html

29. Piller C. FDA and NIH let clinical trial sponsors keep results secret and break the law. *Science*. Published January 13, 2020. https://www.science.org/content/article/ fda-and-nih-let-clinical-trial-sponsors-keep-results-secret-and-break-law

30. U.S. Food & Drug Administration. Office of global operations. Updated December 2021. https://www.fda.gov/about-fda/office-global-policy-and-strategy/office-global-operations

31. Livingston AN, Mattingly TJ 2nd. Drug and medical device product failures and the stability of the pharmaceutical supply chain. *J Am Pharm Assoc*. 2021;61(1):e119-e122. doi:10.1016/j .japh.2020.07.005. https://www.ncbi.nlm.nih.gov/pmc/articles/PMC7395820/

32. Eban K. *Bottle of Lies: The Inside Story of the Generic Drug Boom*. 1st ed. HarperCollins; 2019.

33. Cubanski J, Neuman T, Freed M. What's the latest on Medicare drug price negotiations? *Kaiser Family Foundation*. Published July 23, 2021. https://www.kff.org/medicare/ issue-brief/whats-the-latest-on-medicare-drug-price-negotiations/

34. Carlisle RP, Flint ND, Hopkins ZH, Eliason MJ, Duffin KC, Secrest AM. Administrative burden and costs of prior authorizations in a dermatology department. *JAMA Dermatol*. 2020;156(10):1074-1078. doi:10.1001/jamadermatol.2020.1852

35. Howell S, Yin PT, Robinson JC. Quantifying the economic burden of drug utilization management on payers, manufacturers, physicians, and patients. *Health Affairs*. 2021;40(8). https://www.healthaffairs.org/doi/10.1377/hlthaff.2021.00036?url_ver=Z39.88-2003&rfr_ id=ori:rid:crossref.org&rfr_dat=cr_pub%20%200pubmed

36. Dafny L, Ho K, Kong E. How do copayment coupons affect branded drug prices and quantities purchased? *National Bureau of Economic Research*. Published February 2022. https://www.nber.org/papers/w29735

37. Pacific Research Institute. New brief highlights the economic costs of pharmacy benefit managers.. Published May 8, 2017. https://www.pacificresearch.org/ new-brief-highlights-the-economic-costs-of-pharmacy-benefit-managers/

38. Fein AJ. How GoodRx profits from our broken pharmacy pricing system. *Drug Channels*. Published August 31, 2020. https://www.drugchannels.net/2020/08/how-goodrx-profits-from-our-broken.html

39. Mark Cuban Cost Plus Drug Company. No middlemen. No price games. Huge drug savings. July 2022. www.costplusdrugs.com

40. Lalani HS, Kesselheim AS, Rome BN. Direct-to-consumer generic drugs: a maverick approach or another exposure of market failures? *Ann Intern Med*. 2022;175(6):890-891. doi:10.7326/M22-0740

41. Symbicort/AstraZeneca. What can I expect to pay for SYMBICORT? July 2022. https:// www.mysymbicort.com/cost-assistance.html#:~:text=What%20can%20I%20expect%20 to,(160%2F4.5%20mcg).

42. Hamel L, Lopes L, Kirzinger A, et al. Public opinion on prescription drugs and their prices. *Kaiser Family Foundation*. Polling. Published April 5, 2022. https://www.kff.org/ health-costs/poll-finding/public-opinion-on-prescription-drugs-and-their-prices/

43. Ioannidis JPA. Contradicted and initially stronger effects in highly cited clinical research. *JAMA: J Am Med Assoc*. 2005;294(2):218-228.

44. Ioannidis JPA. Why most published research findings are false. *PLoS Med*. 2005; 2(8):e124.

45. Emerson GB, Warme WJ, Wolf FM, et al. Testing for the presence of positive-outcome bias in peer review: a randomized controlled trial. *Arch Intern Med.* 2010;170(21):1934-1939.

46. Dawn K, Altman DG, Arnaiz JA, et al. Systematic review of the empirical evidence of study publication bias and outcome reporting bias. *PLoS One.* 2008;3(8):e3081.

47. Lexchin J, Bero LA, Djulbegovic B, Clark O. Pharmaceutical industry sponsorship and research outcome and quality: systematic review. *BMJ.* 2003;326(7400):1167-1170.

48. Cousin J, Unger K. Cleaning up the paper trail. *Science.* 2006;312(5770):38-43.

49. Rao TS, Andrade C. The MMR vaccine and autism: sensation, refutation, retraction, and fraud. *Indian J Psychiatry.* 2011;53(2):95-96. doi:10.4103/0019-5545.82529

50. Pharmaceutical Commerce. Sales rep count hold relatively steady at 70,000, says ZS. Published November/December 2017. https://www.pharmaceuticalcommerce.com/view/sales-rep-count-holds-relatively-steady-70000-says-zs

51. ZS. News & Events. Get the latest news, press releases and events. July 2022. https://www.zs.com/about/newsroom/crossing-the-threshold-more-than-half-of-physicians-restrict-access-to-sales-reps

52. Ornstein C, Thomas K. Top cancer researcher fails to disclose corporate financial ties in major research journals. *The New York Times.* Published September 8, 2018. https://www.nytimes.com/2018/09/08/health/jose-baselga-cancer-memorial-sloan-kettering.html?module=inline

53. Fresques H, Jones RG, Ornstein C. How we analyzed Doctors' pharma industry ties and Medicare prescribing. *ProPublica.* Published December 20, 2019. https://projects.propublica.org/graphics/d4dpartd-methodology

54. Adams R. UnitedHealthcare guided Yale's groundbreaking surprise billing study. *The Intercept.* Published August 10, 2021. https://theintercept.com/2021/08/10/unitedhealthcare-yale-surprise-billing-study/

55. Congressional Budget Office. Prescription drugs: spending, use, and prices. Updated January 2022. https://www.cbo.gov/publication/57772

56. Public Citizen. Congress Watch. Rx R&D myths: the case against the drug industry's R&D "Scare Card". Published July 2001. https://www.citizen.org/wp-content/uploads/rdmyths.pdf

57. Wouters OJ, McKee M, Luyten J. Estimated research and development investment needed to bring a new medicine to market, 2009-2018. *JAMA.* 2020;323(9):844-853. doi:10.1001/jama.2020.1166. https://jamanetwork.com/journals/jama/article-abstract/2762311

58. DiMasi JA, Grabowski HG, Hansen RW. Innovation in the pharmaceutical industry: new estimates of R&D costs. J Health Econ. 2016;47: 20-33. https://www.sciencedirect.com/science/article/pii/S0167629616000291?via%3Dihub

59. PhRMA. Biopharmaceutical research & development: the process behind new medicines. July 2022. http://phrma-docs.phrma.org/sites/default/files/pdf/rd_brochure_022307.pdf

60. Schwartz LM, Woloshin S. Medical marketing in the United States, 1997-2016. *JAMA.* 2019;321(1):80-96. doi:10.1001/jama.2018.19320

61. AHIP. New study: in the midst of COVID-19 crisis, 7 out of 10 big pharma companies spent more on sales and marketing than R&D. Published October 27, 2021. https://www.ahip.org/news/articles/new-study-in-the-midst-of-covid-19-crisis-7-out-of-10-big-pharma-companies-spent-more-on-sales-and-marketing-than-r-d

62. Kaiser Family Foundation. Poll: nearly 1 in 4 Americans taking prescription drugs say it's difficult to their medicines, including larger shares among those with health issues, with low incomes and nearing Medicare age. Published March 1, 2019. https://www.kff.org/health-costs/press-release/poll-nearly-1-in-4-americans-taking-prescription-drugs-say-its-difficult-to-afford-medicines-including-larger-shares-with-low-incomes/

63. American Hospital Association. New report shows impact of rising drug prices and drug shortages on patients and hospitals. Published January 15, 2019. https://www.aha.org/press-releases/2019-01-15-new-report-shows-impact-rising-drug-prices-and-drug-shortages-patients

64. Sumarsono A, Lalani HS, Vaduganathan M, et al. Trends in utilization and cost of low-density lipoprotein cholesterol–lowering therapies among Medicare beneficiaries: an analysis from the Medicare part D database. *JAMA Cardiol*. 2021;6(1):92-96. doi:10.1001/jamacardio.2020.3723. https://jamanetwork.com/journals/jamacardiology/fullarticle/2770174

65. Patient-Centered Outcomes Research Institute. What is PCORI's official policy on cost and cost-effectiveness analysis? Accessed July 2022. https://help.pcori.org/hc/en-us/articles/213716587-What-is-PCORI-s-official-policy-on-cost-and-cost-effectiveness-analysis-

66. Angell M. Excess in the pharmaceutical industry. *CMAJ*. 2004;171(12):1451-1453. https://www.cmaj.ca/content/171/12/1451.

67. Angell M. *The Truth About the Drug Companies: How They Deceive Us and What to Do About It*. 1st ed. Random House; 2004.

68. LaMattia J. Even me-too drugs matter when it comes to new medicines. *STAT*. Published September 24, 2021. https://www.statnews.com/2021/09/24/me-too-drugs-matter-when-it-comes-to-new-medicines/

69. Sampat B. The government and pharmaceutical innovation: looking back and looking ahead. *J Law Med Ethics*. 2021;49(1):10-18. doi:10.1017/jme.2021.3

70. Coukell A, Shih C, Reese E. Beyond EpiPen: prices of lifesaving epinephrine products soar. *PEW*. Published September 22, 2016. https://www.pewtrusts.org/en/research-and-analysis/articles/2016/09/22/beyond-epipen-prices-of-lifesaving-epinephrine-products-soar

71. Roberts DK. The deadly costs of insulin. *AJMC*. Published June 11, 2019. https://www.ajmc.com/view/the-deadly-costs-of-insulin

72. Oversight. Drug pricing investigation. Majority staff report. Committee on Oversight and Reform U.S. House of Representatives. Published December 2021. https://oversight.house.gov/sites/democrats.oversight.house.gov/files/DRUG%20PRICING%20REPORT%20WITH%20APPENDIX%20v3.pdf

73. O'Neill Hayes T, Farmer J. Insulin cost and pricing trends. American Action Forum. Published April 2, 2020. https://www.americanactionforum.org/research/insulin-cost-and-pricing-trends/

74. Sable-Smith B. Insulin's high cost leads to lethal rationing. Shots, Health News from NPR. Health Inc. Published September 1, 2018. https://www.npr.org/sections/health-shots/2018/09/01/641615877/insulins-high-cost-leads-to-lethal-rationing

75. Civica. Making insulin affordable for all. Accessed July 2022. https://www.civicainsulin.org/

76. Vincent Rajkumar S. The high cost of prescription drugs: causes and solutions. *Blood Cancer J*. 2020;10:71. doi:10.1038/s41408-020-0338-x

6

Policy

Questions as you read through the chapter:

1. What factors in your everyday life and environment affect your health, and how are those factors determined? How do we decide whether something is "health policy" or not?
2. What laws and elements of health policy have affected you?
3. Who should decide health policy and how should it be decided?
4. Policymakers sometimes move jobs from industry/lobbying to the executive branch administration or Congress, and vice versa. What is good about this? What is bad about this?
5. What values or principles should be upheld in health reform?

Timeline of Major Public Health and Health Policy Developments

1752: First voluntary hospital opens in Philadelphia; New York soon follows.

1777: George Washington orders soldiers to be given smallpox inoculation.

1840s: American Medical Association (AMA) and Pfizer founded

1860s: The Civil War. Development of medical specialties, evidence-based medicine, and the first ambulances

Late 1800s: Development of state and local public health activities, with founding of boards of health, health laboratories, and public health clinics

1906: First Food and Drug Act passed, precursor to the U.S. Food and Drug Administration (FDA)

1910s: World War I. The Flexner Report leads to the creation of modern medical education. Multiple efforts to pass universal health insurance fail.

1929: Baylor Hospital in Texas offers prepaid hospital insurance to a group of teachers as the first insurance plan—this eventually develops into Blue Cross insurance.

1930s: The Great Depression. Birth of the modern Department of Health and Human Services (HHS), FDA, and the National Institutes of Health (NIH). Passage of the Social Security Act. Blue Shield insurance formed to cover physician services

1940s: World War II. Employers offer health insurance to entice workers during wage freeze—birth of modern employee sponsored insurance (ESI).

1946: Passage of the Hill-Burton Act leads to the construction and development of more hospitals and clinics.

1948: President Truman campaigns for national health insurance; it fails.

1951: The Joint Commission founded to improve the quality of hospitals through voluntary accreditation

1950s-60s: Civil Rights era. Federal employees offered health benefits, ESI strengthened with tax benefits, and Indian Health Service formed. Several proposals to include health insurance for Social Security beneficiaries fail.

1965: Medicare and Medicaid programs signed into law; neighborhood health centers established as a precursor to federally qualified health centers (FQHCs)

1970-80s: Gradual expansion of Medicare and Medicaid eligibility. Health spending rises, and Congress starts enacting laws to limit it, including the development of health maintenance organizations (HMOs) and diagnosis-related groups (DRGs). Multiple presidents support national health insurance (Nixon, Carter, Clinton).

1974: Birth of Certificate of Need laws. National Research Act passed to better protect human subjects in research studies

1980: Bayh-Dole Act allows private companies to patent drugs created with publicly funded research.

1984: Hatch-Waxman Act offers drug patents and exclusivity for brand name drugs while also developing an encouraging pathway for the approval of generics.

1985: The Consolidated Omnibus Budget Reconciliation Act (COBRA) passes; offers temporary health coverage for employees who lost their jobs.

1986: The Emergency Medical Treatment and Active Labor Act (EMTALA) passes, requiring hospitals to screen and stabilize patients in the emergency room (ER) regardless of ability to pay.

1990s: Development of electronic medical records, particularly at the Veterans Affairs (VA). Rise of utilization management and HMOs as a cost containment strategy by payers

1990: Americans with Disabilities Act passes. National Committee on Quality Assurance forms to accredit managed care health plans.

1993: President Clinton tries to pass national health insurance; it fails.

1996: The Health Insurance Portability and Accountability Act (HIPAA) passes, setting standards for the privacy of medical records and strengthens some consumer protections in insurance.

1997: Birth of Medicare Advantage (MA)

2003: Birth of Medicare Part D. Development of health savings accounts/flexible spending accounts (HSAs/FSAs)

2006: Massachusetts and Vermont experiment with state-based health reform, aiming for near-universal coverage.

2009: The Health Information Technology for Economic and Clinical Health (HITECH) Act passes, requiring the "meaningful use" of electronic health records (EHRs).

2010: The Affordable Care Act (ACA) passes. Many states refuse to expand Medicaid eligibility.

2015: The Medicare Access and CHIP Reauthorization Act of 2015 (MACRA) passes; changes the way Medicare pays outpatient clinicians.

2010s: Multiple attempts to repeal the ACA fail.

2016: The 21st Century Cures Act passes, aiming to streamline the research and FDA process as well as improve interoperability and give patients their own EHR data.

2020-2021: COVID-19 pandemic. Passage of the two acts, Coronavirus Aid, Relief, and Economic Security (CARES) and American Recovery and Reinvestment Act (ARRA), provided massive financial support to health care institutions and made testing and care for COVID-19 free for patients, including the uninsured. Life expectancy falls, the biggest decline since World War II.

Policy Making in America

To understand how health policy gets made and enacted in America, it's important to consider a few distinctions. Policy can be laws (such as HIPAA), it can be guidelines (such as the CDC's guidance for quarantine after COVID-19 exposures), or regulations enforced by nonlegal consequences from industry organizations (such as losing hospital accreditation from The Joint Commission if you don't follow their regulations). Further, all of these types of policies can come from different levels: local, state, and national. Remember, too, that the government is also an insurer (or purchaser of medical services) and can enforce its codes, rules, and regulations by either reimbursement penalties or by refusing to let a provider participate in its programs.

Who Makes Policy?

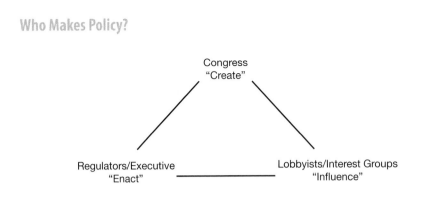

Congress and Legislatures

The U.S. Congress has several committees active in health policy, most notably the Committee on Health, Education, Labor, and Pensions (HELP). Between 2019 and 2021, Congress and the president signed 19 laws related to health.[1] State legislatures have parallel structures. For instance, in 2020, the Missouri legislature passed 18 laws related to health.[2] (For more information on how legislation gets made, we recommend watching the Schoolhouse rock classic, "I'm Just a Bill.")

Executive Branch

Congress and the state legislatures pass laws and the executive branch is charged to enact them. The basic functions of a civil service—that is, the permanent professional branches of the executive branch—devoted to public health are to gather data, communicate information to the public, coordinate as seamlessly as possible with multiple government and community stakeholders, and support policies and laws that promote health.

Federal health administration

The Department of Health and Human Services (HHS) is the primary administrative driver of health policy within the federal government as well as non-health programs, such as Head Start and faith-based and neighborhood partnerships. The HHS is huge, with a budget in 2021 of about $1.3 trillion.[3] (In comparison, the U.S. Department of Defense budget in 2021 was $704 billion,[4] and the total federal budget was $6.8 trillion.[5]) The head of the HHS and the agencies listed subsequently are appointed by the president, whereas the vast majority of the workers in these departments are career employees and technically nonpartisan.[6] Within the umbrella of the HHS are a number of major agencies that affect our daily lives. All of the following have already been discussed throughout the preceding chapters.

Centers for Medicare & Medicaid Services (CMS)—features prominently in Chapters 2 and 3: Medicare is the nation's largest insurer, and as the agency overseeing Medicare and Medicaid, CMS policy is the dominant driver of how—and how much—hospitals and providers get reimbursed. By determining coverage and reimbursement of medical services, drugs, and devices, CMS also has enormous influence on how health care is delivered.

Food and Drug Administration (FDA) —features prominently in Chapter 5: The aim of the FDA is to protect us from the "snake oil" fraudsters of the past, setting a regulatory standard for quality and safety of food products, pharmaceuticals, biologics, medical devices, and veterinary products. Interestingly, the FDA primarily has regulatory influence in the United States, even though the majority of pharmaceuticals and raw materials are manufactured overseas.

National Institutes of Health (NIH) —features prominently in Chapter 5: The NIH is the main government institution responsible for biomedical and health research; it's a major source of funding for medical research in the United States. The NIH awards grants to medical researchers across the country, as well as employing and funding its own research staff. It maintains a number of centers and institutes, including the National Institute of Mental Health and the National Cancer Institute. Dr Anthony Fauci, for instance, became the nation's adviser on COVID-19 because he was the director of a subagency of the NIH, the National Institute of Allergy and Infectious Disease.

*Centers for Disease Control and Prevention (CDC)—*The CDC, headquartered in Atlanta, is the primary agency for public health and epidemiology. It became a household name during the COVID-19 pandemic, but it has enormous reach in many areas, including health promotion (such as exercise recommendations), infectious disease (such as tracking what vaccines travelers should get), and chronic disease (such as tracking the prevalence of type 2 diabetes mellitus).

*Agency for Healthcare Research and Quality (AHRQ)—*This agency gets less press than do the others. The AHRQ oversees health systems and outcomes research (and thus provides a lot of background for this book!). Studies focus on cost, access, and quality of U.S. health care. The AHRQ is a major resource for cataloging clinical practice guidelines, as well.[2]

*Surgeon General—*The surgeon general is the federal government's spokesperson for the nation on matters of health, who often spearheads large public health campaigns, such as encouraging Americans to quit smoking. The surgeon general represents the U.S. government in a number of committees and private organizations and is the head of the Public Health Service Commissioned Corps, which includes 6,000 officers nationwide.

Beyond the HHS, other federal agencies engage in public health projects, such as the Department of Agriculture, Housing and Urban Development, Transportation, and the Environmental Protection Agency.

State and local administration (public health departments)

Much of public health work falls within local and state control, especially administering Medicaid programs and funding. It's difficult to give an overall picture of how this work looks because there is a huge amount of variety in the structure of public health administration from state to state or even county to county within a state. Some local public health agencies and activities started locally before there even was an HHS or a CDC.

Although, historically, public health agencies focused largely on infection control, their scope has expanded over time to include chronic noncommunicable diseases (such as diabetes), preventive health, environmental health, violence and injury prevention, and maternal health, among others. Public health agencies are involved in many elements of everyday life (such as what foods are on offer for school lunches, or what shots you get in the fall), as well as big events such as natural disasters (ie, Hurricane Katrina in 2005) or food poisoning outbreaks (ie, listeria linked to Tyson chicken in 2001). State and local public health agencies also provide some direct clinical care to poor and underserved populations, particularly in the areas of mental illness, tuberculosis, human immunodeficiency virus (HIV)/acquired immunodeficiency syndrome (AIDS), and substance use disorders.

Yet, even as the public health scope has expanded, financing has shrunk. Public health spending in 2018 was just 2.5 cents for every health care dollar.[7] Over the decades before the pandemic, not only did funding decrease (leading to understaffing and rusty surveillance capabilities, worse in some states and counties than in others) but also funding streams were more haphazard, making it difficult to create large-scale and cross-sector projects.[8] This variety combined with underfunding can lead to inefficiency, redundancy, poor coordination, outdated data collection systems, and ineffective action. Many have felt that the COVID-19 pandemic exposed these very weaknesses and have called for a strengthening of the public health infrastructure.

Although the public doesn't have the highest trust in public health institutions (just 52% state they trust the CDC[a]), most—71%—support expanding funding.[9] We are estimated to need $4.5 billion more in funding.[10] Yet, although laws such as the 2020 CARES and the 2021 ARRA each appropriated

---

[a]Which is shockingly low for the biggest public health agency in the nation!

$50 million for public health as part of the pandemic response, neither cre-
ated sustained funding.[8]

Interest Groups

Lobbying is a practice by which businesses, organizations, advocacy groups,
and individuals try to inform and persuade the executive and legislative
branches of federal, state, and local governments to vote or act in ways that
promote or protect certain interests. Lobbyists may influence legislative and
administrative bodies by sponsoring information sessions, helping to draft
legislation, influencing the rules and regulations related to legislation, and
contributing to political campaigns.

You can't talk about interest groups in American health care without
talking about the American Medical Association (AMA). The AMA was
founded in 1847 and is the largest and most powerful professional organization of U.S. physicians. In the 1950s, about 75% of U.S. physicians were members; today, only 15% pay dues.[11] Despite this decline in official membership,
by connecting 170+ specialty societies in its House of Delegates, the AMA acts
like an umbrella organization relevant to most physicians. The AMA remains
a dominant force as a lobbying group as well as in determining physician payment. (No better evidence for this than in the Relative Value Scale Update
Committee [RUC; see page 184] and Current Procedural Terminology [CPT;
see page 75] code books.) The AMA is also known for repeatedly blocking
national health reform measures, including Medicare for All, that the organization hasn't seen as serving the interest of the physicians it represents.

Beyond the AMA, there are dozens of other professional organizations,
trade associations, unions, disease- or identity-specific groups, and think
tanks that shape the politics of health care.

Health-related lobbying accounts for more spending than does almost
any other industry sector, outpacing even defense and energy lobbying.[13] As
you can see from Table 6.1, some pretty large amounts of money get thrown
around. Note that the AMA is not the biggest contributor.

Government Spending: Focus on CMS

From a big picture perspective, the federal government gets money from taxpayers and then spends some of that money on health, largely through the
HHS administration discussed earlier in this chapter. Although some of the
total HHS budget goes toward public health in a broad sense, about 85% of
it flows through CMS to pay for care of Medicare and Medicaid beneficiaries.[12] From a budgetary perspective, the U.S. federal government has been
described as "an insurance company with an army."[13] Although the rise in
health spending as a share of gross domestic product (GDP) is striking, as

Table 6.1 Lobbying Spending

Sector	Total (2020; in million dollars)	Top three contributors (2021; in millions)
Pharmaceuticals and health products	306.2	Pharmaceutical Research and Manufacturers of America: $22.9 Biotechnology Innovation Organization: $9.9 Roche Holding: $9.1
Insurance	151.9	Blue Cross/Blue Shield: $13.4 America's Health Insurance Plans: $8.7 Cigna Corp: $5.8
Hospitals and nursing homes	108.8	American Hospital Association: $17.6 HCA Healthcare: $2.9 Children's Hospital Association: $2.8
Health professionals	87.6	American Medical Association: $14.6 American Academy of Family Physicians: $2.7 American Dental Association: $1.7

Adapted from Statista. Leading lobbying industries in the United States in 2021, by total lobbying spending. https://www.statista.com/statistics/257364/top-lobbying-industries-in-the-us/; Open Secrets. Industries. https://www.opensecrets.org/federal-lobbying/industries

noted in Chapter 3, Figure 6.1 shows the even more dramatic rise of health spending as a percentage of total federal government spending.

CMS makes payments to clinicians, providers, and institutions (hospitals, nursing facilities, laboratories, pharmacies, medical equipment companies … the list goes on) for Medicare beneficiaries, besides paying states for Medicaid beneficiaries.

To understand how that money has been spent in the past—and thus make decisions on how it should be spent in the future—the government relies on several independent, nonpartisan federal agencies. First, the Congressional Budget Office (CBO), founded in 1974, offers detailed and long-range projections on how much policies will cost, and not just in health care. Every time you hear that a bill might cost x or y billions or trillions over the next decade, like the ACA in 2009, the projections were made by the CBO.

Second, there are independent branches evaluating Medicare- and Medicaid-specific spending. The Medicare Payment Advisory Commission (MedPAC) evaluates Medicare, and the Medicaid and CHIP Payment and Access Commission (MACPAC) evaluates Medicaid (you will be forgiven if you mix these acronyms up). MedPAC, founded in 1997, reviews Medicare financing while also commenting on quality and access to care for Medicare

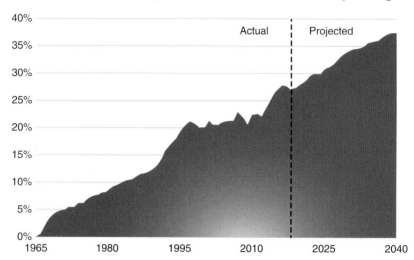

Health Care Spending as a Share of Total Federal Spending

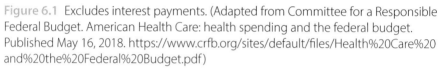

Figure 6.1 Excludes interest payments. (Adapted from Committee for a Responsible Federal Budget. American Health Care: health spending and the federal budget. Published May 16, 2018. https://www.crfb.org/sites/default/files/Health%20Care%20 and%20the%20Federal%20Budget.pdf)

beneficiaries. MACPAC was started in 2009 and does the same for Medicaid. Policy wonks-to-be should look up their free, publicly available, and regularly updated reports online.[b]

Let's look at several major elements of how federal health spending gets determined.

Setting Payments to Physicians,[c] Part 1: the RVU Update Committee (RUC)

(For background on relative value units and fee-for-service, see Section "Understanding Reimbursement" in Chapter 3.) Since the early 1990s, the AMA has operated the RUC, the committee that sets RVU recommendations. The committee comprises 32 physicians, 22 of whom are nominated by specialty societies, representing the array of physician specialties. The committee polls hundreds of physicians to determine the "time and intensity" required for physicians' work. The committee then sends their recommendations to CMS, which historically accepts them over 90% of the time.[14] CMS then independently sets the price paid per RVU (ie, the fee schedule; see Chapter 3) by applying a "conversion factor." For instance, the conversion factor has previously been used to keep reimbursements the same even when RVUs rose.

---

[b]See Suggested Reading.
[c]Here, we use the term *physician* rather than *clinician* because the system is based on payment to physicians. Advanced practice providers are typically paid at a lower rate based on this same system.

Although RVUs are set for CMS, other payers also use them. As such, the RUC (and, by extension, the AMA) holds enormous power over reimbursement for physicians, making it controversial. Some of the arguments both critics and supporters make are provided in Table 6.2.

Setting Payment to Physicians, Part 2: MACRA and the Quality Payment Program

Many physicians would be unable to tell you what the Quality Payment Program (QPP) is or how it works. Let's try to make it as simple as possible. Earlier, we told you about RVUs. Medicare sets the fee schedule for how much money physicians make per RVU. In the late 1980s, policymakers instituted something called a sustainable growth rate (SGR) that tied Medicare expenditures to the rate of overall economic growth. All was well and good until the early 2000s, when the economy worsened, and the SGR would have drastically cut physician payments; given the lobbying power of physician groups, this was a no-go. So every year, Congress would pass a "doc fix" bill to keep physician payments the same. As it turns out, the SGR wasn't so sustainable after all.

Table 6.2 Physician Reimbursement Arguments, Critics Versus Supporters

Critics[14]	Supporters
It makes no sense for physicians to determine their own reimbursement.	They don't set the rates, they set the scale. Physicians can provide the best information about how to value their work relative to each other.
The RUC overrepresents specialties; only five committee members currently represent primary care. The committee thus overvalues specialty procedures, skewing salaries to the detriment of primary care.	The RUC does support primary care, including advocating for increased valuation of non-procedural services, preventive services, and chronic care management.[15] Because it's a zero-sum game, this means the valuation has shifted away from specialty/procedural care.
The RUC is too secretive and lacks sufficient oversight to ensure that its recommendations impact the overall good of the system rather than being self-interested.	The RUC has increased transparency of their discussions and recommendations over time.[16] CMS has adequate oversight in its discretion to accept or not accept recommendations.

CMS, Centers for Medicare & Medicaid Services; RUC, Relative Value Scale Update Committee.
Adapted from Goodson JD. Unintended consequences of resource-based relative value scale reimbursement. *JAMA*. 2007;298(19):2308-2310. doi:10.1001/jama.298.19.2308; The American Medical Association/Specialty Society RVS Update Committee's long history of improving payment for primary care services. Updated May 2022. https://www.ama-assn.org/system/files/2019-02/ruc-primary-care.pdf; AMA/Specialty Society RVS Update Committee significant process improvements—2012/2013. https://www.ama-assn.org/sites/ama-assn.org/files/corp/media-browser/public/rbrvs/improvements-to-ruc_0.pdf

In 2015, the SGR was replaced with the Medicare Access and CHIP Reauthorization Act of 2015 (MACRA). MACRA tied physician payments not to economic growth but instead to quality measures, through the QPP. This applies primarily to physicians who bill enough to Medicare Part B (so, outpatient care, not inpatient care). Physicians have two options in the QPP, both of which are moving toward alternative payment models (APMs): take part in the Merit-based Incentive Payment System (MIPS) or take on risk as part of an APM. MIPS itself is a step toward being an APM, scoring categories of performance (such as quality and cost) and adjusting physician payments with bonuses or penalties. Both MIPS and APMs require use of EHRs, documentation of various measures, and complicated algorithms for adjusting payments.

Increasingly, Medicaid and private insurance are instituting their own forms of MIPS-like payment adjustments, for instance, the Quality Incentive Program in Managed Medicaid programs.

Enough acronyms for you? The big take-aways here are as follows:

1. Medicare is increasingly making moves away from FFS reimbursements and toward quality, or value-based, payments. In fact, CMS states a goal of moving *all* beneficiaries into APMs by 2030[17] (see Section "APMs and Value-Based Payment" in Chapter 3).
2. The complicated nature of this policy—far, far more complicated than what we've distilled here—means that many physicians either rely on their health system to figure this out or rely on contracting vendors to do it for them. Elsewhere in this book, we talk about the high cost of health care administration [see Section "Why Does U.S. Health Care Cost So Much?" in Chapter 3], the burden of sometimes bad quality metrics [see Section "Choosing the Right Metrics" in Chapter 4], and the shift of physicians from independent practitioners to employees [see Section "Networks and Consolidation" in Chapter 2]. Such a context has to be considered even in the important transition to paying for "value over volume."[d]

Setting Payments to States in Medicaid: Federal Medical Assistance Program

Medicaid is a joint federal-state partnership. The federal government gives a variable amount of money to states on the basis of how much that state spends (basically, a matching payment), as well as formulas accounting for the per capita income of the state (ie, poorer states get more money). This payment to the states, the Federal Medical Assistance Program (FMAP), pays at least 50% and up to 83% of costs.[18]

---

[d]In 2017, even MedPAC, the advisory board comment in Medicare policy, recommended getting rid of the QPP in their annual report!

The government can also increase the FMAP for certain activities as an incentive to states. For instance, when the ACA expanded Medicaid eligibility, they also increased the FMAP for these newly eligible patients to 100% until 2016. So states that expanded eligibility did not have to pay for the newly eligible patients at all in the beginning, offering reassurance against concerns that states would be hurt by rising spending. (States that didn't expand eligibility got no extra money.)

In another example, in 2021, the American Rescue Plan, responding in part to the risks people face in nursing homes (as well as years of advocacy), temporarily increased the FMAP to states that improve their programs for home- and community-based services for seniors and people with disabilities.

Alternatively, Republican reform plans frequently seek to change the FMAP into a "block grant," meaning that each state gets a fixed amount of money only—and thus has an incentive to reduce their spending and enrollment. The Trump Administration was making moves toward block grants before the 2020 election (see Section "Reform" in this chapter on page 189).

Paying for Managed Care: Medicare Advantage (MA) and Managed Medicaid

Traditional or regular Medicare and Medicaid involves direct payments to providers for their services (ie, FFS). Both also include substantial programs of "managed care" (ie, using utilization management tactics, such as an HMO; see Chapter 2), in which a private, nongovernmental insurance plan is paid by CMS to handle costs and care for a group of beneficiaries.

In Medicare, this managed care is contracted out to private, nongovernmental payers, called *Medicare Advantage*, through Part C. MA is an increasing and controversial area of CMS spending, now covering 48% of Medicare patients and accounting for 52% of all Medicare dollars.[19] Although the goal in starting MA was to use competition among private payers to increase quality and decrease costs for Medicare patients, it's not clear that these goals have been met. For example, per-beneficiary spending is rising faster in MA than for traditional Medicare[20]; see Section "Medicare Advantage" in Chapter 3.

Medicaid, too, has managed care; in fact, it's even more prevalent. As of 2018, nearly 70% of Medicaid beneficiaries were in a risk-based managed plan, similar to MA plans, and 46% of Medicaid spending went to these plans.[21]

Paying for Innovation: CMS Innovation Center

The ACA established the Center for Medicare and Medicaid Innovation (CMMI) under CMS, in 2010, allocating $10 billion per decade. CMMI tests out APMs (see Chapter 3), with the long-term goal of lowering spending while improving or maintaining quality. Some of those pilot models are shown in Figure 6.2.

Although CMMI offers exciting opportunities for experimentation in the shift to value-based care, so far the cost savings haven't borne out. CMMI is projected to save money by 2026 (the CBO estimates $34 million; an independent

Financial Performance of CMS Innovation (CMMI) Payment Models

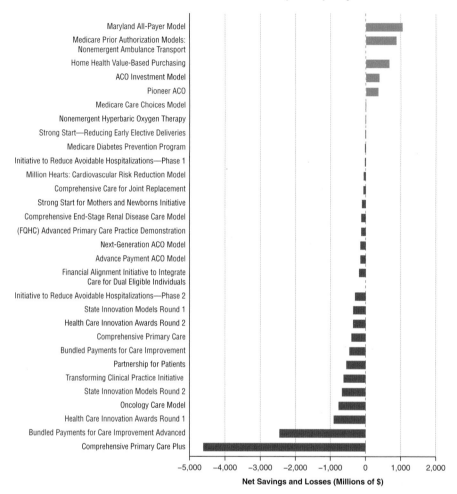

Figure 6.2 Adapted from Smith B. CMS Innovation Center at 10 years—progress and lessons learned. *N Engl J Med.* 2021;384(8):759-764. doi: 10.1056/NEJMsb2031138

consultant estimates a more conservative $18 million in savings[22]), but there has been no noticeable savings to date—in fact, only 5 out of 40 projects have generated savings[23] so far. Experience with CMMI models serves as a reminder that the planned transition from FFS to APMs may make good sense—yet could still be plagued by difficulty and missteps. Figuring out a new way of reimbursing care is pretty complicated to enact, and, of course, value-based payments are subject to attempts to game the system like any other reimbursement mechanism. Further, even regulatory improvements—say, in how risk adjustment is handled—may not be a comprehensive solution to the problems with quality and cost in U.S. health care (see Section "Why Does U.S. Health Care Cost So Much?" in Chapter 3).

Reform

Although reform is happening all the time (such as laws tackling surprise billing, see Section "Surprise Billing"), "health care reform" usually refers to legislation attempting to improve insurance access and decrease cost for large numbers of people. That's what we'll talk about in the following section.

Reform Is Hard

Health care reform has a long, convoluted, messy history in the United States. There has never been one law or coherent system that you could point to and say, "*this* is U.S. health policy," or even, "*this* is what should be reformed." A number of attempts at passing some form of universal insurance coverage have failed, as you can see in the timeline at the beginning of this chapter, and of the two biggest health care laws—the creation of Medicare in 1965 and the passing of the ACA in 2010—the latter just barely passed. Given that health care is a large sector of the economy and a major source of jobs, any potential reform will have massive impacts. There are so many stakeholders in U.S. health care— citizens, patient groups, health care workers, hospitals, payers, corporations, employers, manufacturers, unions, and so on—which clamor for laws that will benefit them and try to block those that won't. So, most health policy has been enacted little by little, sometimes nationally and sometimes just in a single state. Because of this patchwork nature, what U.S. health care looks like, and the desirability of its reform, depends a lot on who you are, what you do, where you live, and how happy you are with your current health care benefits.

Although it is very difficult to pass large-scale federal health care legislation through Congress, those who desire reform on the level of the states have options. Hawaii enacted near-universal coverage in 1974. And after national reform efforts failed during the 1990s, several other states took on reform, most notably Vermont and Massachusetts (whose "Romneycare" in 2006 became the model for the ACA). And Maryland, although it does not have universal coverage, does have an independent board that streamlines statewide hospital reimbursements (the same no matter the provider or payer) through its All-Payer Model.

But passing large-scale health care legislation through states is also hard. An easier locus of control is to expand coverage and benefits through Medicaid. The federal government can do this by expanding the FMAP (just as the American Rescue Plan did temporarily in 2021), or by expanding eligibility (as with the ACA). A state can go further by choosing to expand eligibility beyond what's required, or to offer more generous coverage through Medicaid in their state (Massachusetts is again an example).

On the flip side, in opposition to federal involvement in health insurance, some states opt to reform health care by *limiting* Medicaid, through work requirements (attempted in Arkansas) or block grants (ie, giving each state a fixed amount rather than a percentage based on state spending). Other tactics have outright opposed Medicaid expansion reforms. After the Supreme Court determined in 2012 that the ACA could only incentivize rather than mandate Medicaid expansion, only 26 states immediately expanded coverage, and by the end of 2021, 13 states still haven't expanded their Medicaid coverage. Perhaps the most extreme historical example of state opposition to federal reform comes from Arizona, which did not offer Medicaid *at all* to its population until 1982, a full 17 years after Medicaid was enacted (the state was finally swayed by its own county governments and hospitals, which were shouldering the cost of Medicaid-eligible patients). Interestingly, Arizona was one of the few Republican-led states to expand Medicaid in 2014.

Health reform sometimes moves beyond the legislatures to the citizens as a ballot initiative. A few of those states whose governors or legislatures declined to expand Medicaid coverage later did so because the state's citizens wanted it enough that they put it on the ballot and voted for it. This happened in Maine, Idaho, Utah, Nebraska, Oklahoma, and, most recently, in Missouri. Yet even here, different interests can block each other: Missouri voters passed Medicaid expansion through the ballot in 2021, but their state legislature then refused to fund it. (Legal battles are ongoing as of the publishing of this book.)

And some states and citizens have taken universal coverage into their own hands. As of 2021, three states have passed laws offering a public option (see Section "Public Option" in this chapter on page 194); the first, Cascade Select in Washington State, began enrolling beneficiaries in 2021. Colorado and Nevada have also passed some form of a public option, and these are set to take effect later in the 2020s.[24] At least 16 other states were considering something similar—including allowing anyone to purchase Medicaid.[25]

Few would argue that the current U.S. health care (non)system is the best one possible—more like a house that keeps getting new rooms and additions done by different architects and builders—yet, even when everyone wants something done, we can't get anything done. Time and again, reform efforts are blocked. To understand any individual reform effort, we can think of the following framework of questions:

1. Reforming *what* exactly? (Cost? Access? Quality?)
2. Who would the reform help, and who might perceive it as hurting them? (Who gets more money, and who gets less? Does it make the system more or less complex?)
3. What is the distribution of power in the present system, and how would reform change that? (Does it expand the power of the government or private companies?)

4. What is a *goal* (ie, a principle or value, such as universal coverage) of reform, and what is a *mechanism of change*? (What specific things are you changing to meet your goal, such as transitioning from many payers to a single payer?)
5. What ideologies shape different visions or goals of reform?
6. How might ideologies and financial interests create opposition on mechanisms of change even when there's agreement on goals?
7. How might a mechanism of change serve one goal while harming another?

   If you are interested in the history and politics of reform, we highly recommend reading Paul Starr (see Suggested Reading).

Legacy of the ACA at 10 Years

The ACA was passed in 2010, and its provisions took effect by 2014. Immediately, its opponents attempted to weaken and repeal it. Many lawsuits went through the courts, even getting to the Supreme Court in 2012 and 2021. Repeal attempts sped through a Republican Congress, with over 50 unsuccessful bills from 2010 to 2016 while Obama was still president.[26] In 2017, under a Republican president with a Republican Congress, three repeal-and-replace bills failed. Amid all these failures, Congress, the Supreme Court, and a Republican executive branch did change some provisions, altering the law from its original intentions. Having withstood all these efforts, it now seems the ACA, or "Obamacare," is here to stay.

So, after a decade, what is the ACA's legacy? We'll do our best to summarize in five categories what the impact of this 2000+ page law has been over the past decade.

- **Consumer Protections:** As discussed in Section "What Did the ACA Change About Insurance Coverage (Mostly)?" in Chapter 2, now insurance must offer the same basic premium costs as well as basic coverage to each person, cover young adults up to age 26 on their parents' insurance, can't deny you for a preexisting condition, and won't impose lifetime limits on what they'll pay for you. Beyond this, the Marketplaces serve as a trustworthy forum in which to compare different plans, reducing the likelihood of a patient getting scammed. These consumer protections are very popular and the negative impact of potentially losing them is likely the main reason why repeal could never get off the ground.
- **Reinforcing Incrementalism:** The ACA expanded coverage by dribs and drabs—expanding Medicaid here, requiring employers to offer insurance there, and so on—rather than a sweeping reform that covered everyone.

This reinforced the patchwork nature of the current insurance system, and made continued incrementalism the easiest path for future reforms.

- **Entrenching ESI:** Tying health insurance to employment has significant downsides, and many wanted to scrap it. Instead, it was an important strategy in incrementalism. For better or for worse, the ACA reinforced ESI for the long term.

- **Shifting to Value:** The ACA tied hospital and provider FFS reimbursement to quality and cost in a number of ways, launched new value-based alternative payment models such as ACOs, and created CMMI to test innovative models. This trend of reimbursement based on *value* rather than on *volume* has only grown in the past decade and will likely eclipse FFS in the future.

- **Insuring an Extra 20 Million[27]:** The expansion of Medicaid accounted for over half of that additional coverage.[28] The private insurance industry also saw an overall 6.2% rise in revenue because of increased enrollment.[29,e] Despite the significant insurance expansions, 29 million people remain uninsured (Figure 6.3; see Section "No Insurance" in Chapter 2).

- **Spending:** Medicare spending increased, but at 20% lower than projected.[30] Medicaid expansion cost the federal government an extra $128 billion.[28]

Uninsured Rate Among the Nonelderly Population, 1972-2018

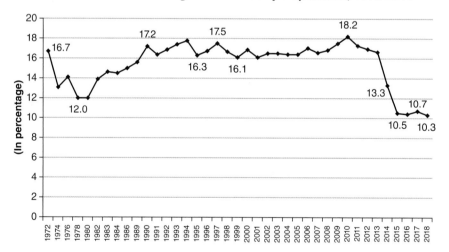

Figure 6.3 Note: 2018 data are for Q1 only. (Adapted from Kaiser Family Foundation. Uninsured rate among the nonelderly population, 1972-2018. Published August 28, 2018. https://www.kff.org/uninsured/slide/uninsured-rate-among-the-nonelderly-population-1972-2018/)

---

[e]However, this premium increase was generally offset by other losses attributable to the ACA.

Many of the cost-cutting measures of the law ended up being postponed or eliminated.[31] Still, overall, most believe the ACA bent the cost curve: Although spending still increased, it increased more slowly than it had before. By 2017, the ACA was estimated to have saved $2.3 trillion than if it had never been passed.[32]

- **Health Outcomes**: This is an extremely difficult assessment to make—and too nuanced to delve into in this introductory text—but most likely some outcomes improved as we might expect from access to insurance (see Chapter 2). Some project that the lack of Medicaid expansion in some states led to over 15,000 preventable deaths.[33]

Understanding Other Reform Options

There are a lot of proposals and potential proposals out there, but all of them fit within one of the following general buckets.

Socialized Medicine

The term *socialized medicine* gets thrown around a lot. Technically, it refers to a system in which the government completely controls both the financing and delivery of health care; the classic example is the National Health Service in the United Kingdom. Within the United States, the VA is also an example of socialized medicine. And, while it's on the private market, Kaiser Permanente is another example of combining financing with delivery (see Chapter 2). There have been no serious national proposals for such a system in the United States.

Single Payer

In a single-payer system, the government would insure everybody and thus control health financing, without controlling delivery. A single-payer system would maintain all of the same provider and hospital systems but would transform the insurance and reimbursement system. The idea is to cover everybody, while slashing the profit motive, administrative costs (by getting rid of redundancy), and high prices (through increased bargaining power). This system would be similar to those of Canada, Japan, Singapore, and Taiwan. Note that all of these systems allow for supplemental private insurance on top of the universal public insurance; for instance, two-thirds of Canadians also have additional private insurance.[34]

"Medicare for All" or M4A is a single-payer proposal; under such a proposal, every American citizen would become eligible for Medicare. However, it's worth remembering that (a) Medicare is far from free and (b) 48% of Medicare patients are in a private insurance plan contracted through MA—neither of these are touted by M4A plans, meaning these reform proposals include changes to the details of Medicare itself, not just expanding eligibility.

Public Option

Proponents of a public option support a government-run insurance system that coexists with private insurance, where citizens have a right to public insurance. Systems that use this model—such as Germany, France, Spain, and Switzerland—can be fairly varied in the details. One way that's been proposed in the United States would be to allow citizens of any age to enroll in Medicare, that is, "Medicare for all who want it." A public option was initially Obama's preference for health reform, but it wasn't politically feasible enough to make it to the ACA. In most countries with public insurance, there are still those who choose to purchase private insurance; in Germany, 11% of citizens are covered by private health insurance.[35] As of 2021, as mentioned on page 190, Washington State became the first state to offer a public option.

Universal Health Coverage

Universal coverage—that is, every citizen has a right to health insurance—is a goal rather than a mechanism, and it is a key component of all of the three systems mentioned earlier. We mention universal coverage separately here only to recognize that there are many mechanisms to achieve this goal. (Remember #4 in our list of framework questions on page 190?) Technically, the U.S. system could achieve universal coverage through enough patchwork options—which is what Democrats such as Presidents Obama and Biden aimed to do, first through the ACA and then by expanding upon the ACA—however, using the rest of the world as an example, it seems impossible to achieve universal coverage without a strong public option. A good example is Singapore, which has public-sponsored basic insurance for all, public-sponsored FSAs to help with out-of-pocket costs, and more robust public insurance for the needy; however, beyond this they require out-of-pocket payments and supplemental private insurance.[36]

Tax Benefits, Incentives, and Insurance Reforms

These are proposals—that is, "mechanisms of change"—that may have different goals: some to expand coverage, some to improve care, some to reduce government role in health care, and others to increase it.

Many proponents of using tax benefits and other incentives want to limit or even decrease the government's role. Major proposals are exemplified in President Trump's bill Healthcare Reform to Make America Great Again, including making the tax breaks on ESI (ie, the money spent on insurance isn't taxed) available for anyone who purchases insurance, allowing insurance to be sold across state lines, and transitioning federal payments to states for Medicaid to block grants (which give only a set amount of funding per state). These were both elements of multiple Repeal-and-Replace plans under a Republican Congress and President Trump, which ultimately did not pass.

Some reform mechanisms are already in use on a small scale, including attempts to use "skin in the game" to lower spending. For instance, since 2007, Indiana has offered both a high-deductible insurance plan plus a flexible spending account (FSA) (see Chapter 2) to state employees, with the state putting some of the deductible amount into the FSA. The idea is for employees to be protected from high costs if needed but incentivized to try lower spending—because they get to keep what isn't spent. Indiana has piloted a similar program for Medicaid beneficiaries since 2011.

In 2021, the Heartland Institute proposed the American Health Plan,[37] which would make direct payments to primary care, eliminate the ACA Marketplaces, disincentivize employer-sponsored insurance, split Medicaid into a long-term program for those with disabilities plus a short-term program primarily covering children, and heavily support new "Health Ownership Accounts," which would operate very similarly to FSAs. This plan would also allow insurers to deny coverage based on preexisting conditions.

Public Opinion

In general, with polling, a lot depends on how a question is asked. Yet, proponents of various ideologies or reforms want to use polling data to show that their proposals are popular and thus should be enacted. So, we should always look at polls with a healthy dose of questioning and skepticism … that being said, here is some polling data.

First, let's ask how Americans view the ACA as a whole (Figure 6.4).

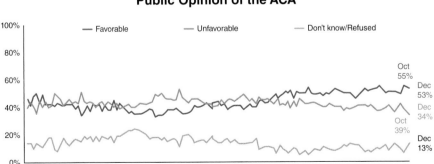

Public Opinion of the ACA

Figure 6.4 Adapted from Kirzinger A, Montero A, Hamel L, Brodie M. 5 charts about public opinion on the Affordable Care Act. *Kaiser Family Foundation*. Published April 14, 2022. https://www.kff.org/health-reform/poll-finding/5-charts-about-public-opinion-on-the-affordable-care-act-and-the-supreme-court/

And how do they view the ACA's individual provisions? (Figure 6.5; hint: people like more benefits.)

The ACA included expansion of both public and private insurance programs. What do Americans think specifically about the government's role in health coverage? (Figure 6.6.)

Most Say It Is Important That ACA Provisions Remain in Place

Percent who say it is "very important" that each of these parts of the ACA is kept in place:	Total	Democrats	Independents	Republicans
Prohibits health insurance companies from denying coverage for people with preexisting conditions	72%	88%	73%	62%
Prohibits health insurance companies from denying coverage to pregnant women	71	89	73	49
Prohibits health insurance companies from charging sick people more	64	76	64	55
Requires health insurance companies to cover the cost for most preventive services	62	80	58	49
Prohibits health insurance companies from setting a lifetime limit	62	72	65	48
Give states the option of expanding their Medicaid programs	57	84	55	36
Provides financial help to low- and moderate-income Americans to help them purchase coverage	57	82	54	31
Prohibits private health insurance companies from setting an annual limit	51	67	46	38
Allows young adults to stay on their parents' insurance plans until age 26	51	68	50	36

Figure 6.5 ACA, Affordable Care Act. (Adapted from Kirzinger A, Montero A, Hamel L, Brodie M. 5 charts about public opinion on the Affordable Care Act. *Kaiser Family Foundation*. Published April 14, 2022. https://www.kff.org/health-reform/poll-finding/5 -charts-about-public-opinion-on-the-affordable-care-act-and-the-supreme-court/)

SOURCE: KFF Health Tracking Poll (conducted July 18-23, 2019). See topline for full question wording and response options.

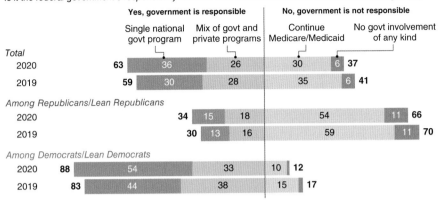

Is it the federal government's responsibility to make sure all Americans have health care coverage? (%)

	Yes, government is responsible		No, government is not responsible	
	Single national govt program	Mix of govt and private programs	Continue Medicare/Medicaid	No govt involvement of any kind

Total
2020 — 63 | 36 | 26 | 30 | 6 | 37
2019 — 59 | 30 | 28 | 35 | 6 | 41

Among Republicans/Lean Republicans
2020 — 34 | 15 | 18 | 54 | 11 | 66
2019 — 30 | 13 | 16 | 59 | 11 | 70

Among Democrats/Lean Democrats
2020 — 88 | 54 | 33 | 10 | 12
2019 — 83 | 44 | 38 | 15 | 17

Note: No answer responses not shown.

Figure 6.6 Note: No answer responses not shown. (Used with permission from Jones B. Increasing share of Americans favor a single government program to provide health care coverage. *Pew Research Center*. Published September 29, 2020. https://www.pewresearch.org/fact-tank/2020/09/29/increasing-share-of-americans-favor-a-single-government-program-to-provide-health-care-coverage/)

That's a lot of people across the political spectrum who not only view the government as responsible for ensuring universal coverage (a goal) but who also seem to think the government programs (a mechanism) are important.

Next, do Americans support expanding Medicare, including Medicare for All? (Figure 6.7.)

How does support change based on context? (Figure 6.8.)

Public's Attitude on Proposals to Expand Medicare and Medicaid

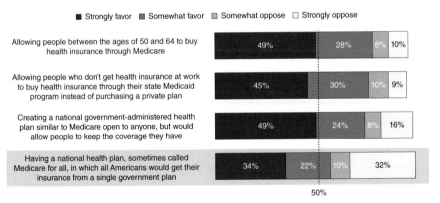

■ Strongly favor ■ Somewhat favor ▨ Somewhat oppose ☐ Strongly oppose

Allowing people between the ages of 50 and 64 to buy health insurance through Medicare — 49% | 28% | 8% | 10%

Allowing people who don't get health insurance at work to buy health insurance through their state Medicaid program instead of purchasing a private plan — 45% | 30% | 10% | 9%

Creating a national government-administered health plan similar to Medicare open to anyone, but would allow people to keep the coverage they have — 49% | 24% | 8% | 16%

Having a national health plan, sometimes called Medicare for all, in which all Americans would get their insurance from a single government plan — 34% | 22% | 10% | 32%

50%

Figure 6.7 Adapted from Kirzinger A, Muñana C, Brodie M. KFF health tracking poll—January 2019: the public on next steps for the ACA and proposals to expand coverage. *Kaiser Family Foundation*. Published January 23, 2019. https://www.kff.org/health-reform/poll-finding/kff-health-tracking-poll-january-2019/?utm_source=link_newsv9&utm_campaign=item_257711&utm_medium=copy

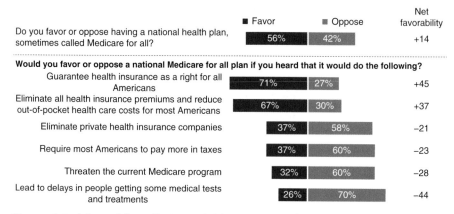

Figure 6.8 Adapted from Kirzinger A, Muñana C, Brodie M. KFF health tracking poll—January 2019: the public on next steps for the ACA and proposals to expand coverage. *Kaiser Family Foundation*. Published January 23, 2019. https://www.kff.org/health-reform/poll-finding/kff-health-tracking-poll-january-2019/?utm_source=link_newsv9&utm_campaign=item_257711&utm_medium=copy

What can we take from all this? In the words of Frank Newport, a scientist for the polling organization Gallup, "Americans have a basic willingness to consider the *idea* of an expansive government-run health system—particularly if it is seen as an extension of the existing Medicare program. But that support appears to be contingent on addressing underlying concerns about the implications of a new system for existing private health care coverage."[38] People like the goal—but they don't want any mechanisms of change to threaten their current benefits.

Hot Button Policy Issues Beyond Large-Scale Reform

Here, we'll go through three issues have been big news; each ties together themes discussed in the delivery, payment, pharmaceutical, research, and quality sections of this book.

Surprise Billing

Surprise billing is when you are seen at an in-network (see Chapter 2) hospital, but you also get an out-of-network bill from a physician whom your insurance has excluded from its network. Such billing can happen even if you had no option to get an in-network physician instead; for instance, if you were at an in-network hospital where, unbeknownst to you, all of the ER physicians are out of network.[f,g] Patients can be hit with huge out-of-network bills (think upward of $100,000![39]), and the practice of surprise billing has been increasing in the past decade. A Yale research team[h] found, for instance, that 11% of anesthesiologists sent surprise bills.[40] The same team found that ending surprise billing would reduce employer-sponsored insurance spending by $40 billion annually. At its heart, this issue shines a light on two things: (a) the chaotic system of contract negotiations between payers and physicians, which the rise of narrow networks and private equity seems to be worsening, and (b) the total lack of transparency or power for patients in this system.

At the beginning of 2022, the No Surprises Act[41] took effect. This law bans surprise billing in some cases (such as anesthesiology care), and reins in out-of-network billing otherwise, including creating a federal mediator system to decide price disputes between insurers and physicians. This law was challenged by lawsuits in 2021—first by the Texas Medical Association[42] and then by the even bigger lobbying groups of the AMA and the American Hospital Association—all focused on the power balance of the mediator system. These interest groups claim that the law favors insurers over providers. The pushback from interest groups underscores the need to assess for changes in shifting power balance in reform measures (see our framework of questions about reform, page 190). It also reminds us that, in health policy, every dollar you save cuts a dollar from someone's paycheck (see Section "Why Does U.S. Health Care Cost So Much?" in Chapter 3).

The Opioid Epidemic

In the mid-20th century, the U.S. government listed opioids on the list of controlled substances (ie, illegal without a prescription), and the use of prescription opioid medications, even for pain control, was severely curtailed. Then, in the 1990s, a movement to better address pain took off, opiate prescriptions for pain were encouraged by clinical experts, and pharmaceutical companies heartily signed on to this trend as they marketed so-called nonaddictive opiates such as OxyContin. By 2017, 191 million opioid prescriptions were dispensed nationwide, with the highest prescribing rate in Alabama and the lowest in Hawaii.[43]

Although only a small percentage of those taking chronic prescription opiates develop addiction, rising prescriptions still helped fuel a crisis of addiction and overdose. Although opioid prescribing peaked in 2010, current prescribing

---

[f]This is unbeknownst to those treating physicians, too, by the way.
[g]Balance billing is slightly different: the provider or hospital charges you directly when they don't think your insurance has paid enough.
[h]See this research mentioned in Section "Conflict of Interest" in Chapter 5.

remains triple what it was in the 1990s[44]—and about 28% of overdose deaths are attributed to prescription opiates.[45] In 2019, 50,000 people died from opioid overdoses in the United States.[46] In 2020, more than twice as many people died from drug overdoses than from COVID-19 in San Francisco.[47]

To combat this, there have been a number of lawsuits and policy changes. Purdue Pharmaceuticals, the makers of OxyContin, was dissolved and paid $4.5 billion to settle opioid-related lawsuit claims.[48] Every state now tracks controlled prescriptions electronically; in California, prescribers are required to check this database once every 4 months for each patient they prescribe controlled substances for. By 2018, most states had enacted laws limiting opioid prescribing.[49] Yet, some worry that laws limiting prescribing may actually fuel the crisis, by driving those with pain toward less-safe illegal options. Addiction medicine experts focus on other policies better aimed at reducing opioid deaths, such as relaxing the licensing requirements for clinicians to prescribe the addiction treatment buprenorphine, as the government did in 2021, and by creating supervised drug-injection sites, as New York did in 2021.[50]

Aduhelm Controversy

Alzheimer dementia is a debilitating disease affecting six million Americans and costing society an extra approximately $216,500 per person with Alzheimer's.[51] Every level of the *Ecology of Medical Care* (see Chapter 1) is involved in dementia management—very much including uncompensated home care—and much research is devoted not only to preventing dementia but also to improving our quality of care for patients with it. Enter Aduhelm (generic name aducanumab), a monoclonal antibody drug manufactured by Biogen. Aduhelm was approved by the FDA in 2021 to treat Alzheimer's—amid a huge outcry against it, including by the FDA's own clinical advisory board. Why? In a nutshell, because of the following reasons:

1. Dementia researchers and experts say the evidence shows aducanumab doesn't provide clinical benefit.[52,53] That is, there is evidence that aducanumab reduces amyloid—the protein buildup that causes Alzheimer's— but not that this amyloid reduction meaningfully improves cognitive ability, functionality, or quality of life (see Section "What are the types of research, and how do they get done?" in Chapter 5).
2. Aduhelm costs a ton of money, $28,000 per patient per year.[54] (Initially, the price was $56,000, but Biogen cut the price in half in response to public outcry. A good example of how pharmaceutical companies set prices as high as they think they can get.[i])

---

[i]See Section "Drug Pricing Controversies" in Chapter 5.

3. So many simpler things that could help dementia patients—in-home care, medical equipment needs, nursing home care, transportation, and so on— are not covered by Medicare.

Some FDA researchers felt so strongly about the FDA decision that they re- signed from the FDA in protest,[55] and many neurologists and geriatricians have voiced their criticism. Others—like the CEO of the Alzheimer's Association— are less critical of the FDA decision but more concerned with the price and resulting risk of (further increasing) inequity for those who cannot access it.[56]

Aduhelm also drove up Medicare premiums in 2022. This is because the 2022 premiums had to be set before any decision by CMS about whether Aduhelm would be covered. Aduhelm, as an injectable drug administered at hospitals or physicians' offices, would have been covered under Medicare Part B. Part B premiums go up most years, but about 50% of the rise in 2022 was due to anticipating how many patients would end up getting this one expensive drug.[57] Instead, Medicare will cover Aduhelm only for beneficiaries using it as part of clinical trials, so a pretty limited number of people. Will this decision set a precedent for Medicare—and potentially for other payers—to determine whether medications are not clinically effective enough to cover, even when the FDA has approved them?

References

1. GovTrack. Health. https://www.govtrack.us/congress/bills/subjects/health/6130#congress =116&current_status[]=28

2. Missouri Foundation for Health. 2022 legislative session. https://mffh.org/our-focus/ policy/legislative-updates/

3. U.S. Department of Health & Human Services. HHS FY 2021 budget in brief. https://www .hhs.gov/about/budget/fy2021/index.html

4. U.S. Department of Defense. DOD releases fiscal year 2021 budget proposal. Published February 10, 2020. https://www.defense.gov/News/Releases/Release/Article/2079489/ dod-releases-fiscal-year-2021-budget-proposal/

5. Congressional Budget Office. Budget. 2022. https://www.cbo.gov/topics/budget

6. Smith RR. Political donations and federal employees in 2020 elections. *FedSmith*. Pub- lished February 12, 2021. https://www.fedsmith.com/2021/02/12/political-donations-and- federal-employees/

7. Green T, Venkataramani AS. Trade-offs and policy options—using insights from economics to inform public health policy. *N Engl J Med*. 2022;386(5):405-408. doi:10.1056/NEJMp2104360

8. Trust for American's Health. The impact of chronic underfunding on America's public health system: Trends, Risks, and Recommendations, 2021. Published May 2021. https:// www.tfah.org/wp-content/uploads/2021/05/2021_PHFunding_Fnl.pdf

9. Harvard TH. The public's perspective on the United States public health system. RWJF/ Harvard School of Public Health. Published May 2021. https://www.rwjf.org/en/library/ research/2021/05/the-publics-perspective-on-the-united-states-public-health-system.html

10. Maani N, Galea S. COVID-19 and underinvestment in the public health infrastructure of the United States. *The Milbank Quarterly*. (Volume 98). Published June 2020. https://www .milbank.org/quarterly/articles/covid-19-and-underinvestment-in-the-public-health-infrastructure-of-the-united-states/#_ednref8

11. Collier R. American Medical Association membership woes continue. *CMAJ*. 2011;183(11): E713-E714. doi:10.1503/cmaj.109-3943

12. Department of Health and Human Services. Putting America's health first FY 2020 President's budget for HHS. https://www.hhs.gov/sites/default/files/fy-2020-budget-in-brief.pdf

13. The Tax-Cut Con. *New York Times*. Published September 14, 2003. http://pkarchive.org/ economy/TaxCutCon.html

14. Goodson JD. Unintended consequences of resource-based relative value scale reimbursement. *JAMA*. 2007;298(19):2308-2310. doi:10.1001/jama.298.19.2308

15. The American Medical Association/Specialty Society RVS Update Committee's long history of improving payment for primary care services. Updated May 2022. https://www .ama-assn.org/system/files/2019-02/ruc-primary-care.pdf

16. AMA/Specialty Society RVS Update Committee significant process improvements— 2012/2013. https://www.ama-assn.org/sites/ama-assn.org/files/corp/media-browser/public/ rbrvs/improvements-to-ruc_0.pdf

17. Centers for Medicare & Medicaid Services. Driving health system transformation—a strategy for the CMS innovation center's second decade. In: *Innovation Center Strategy Refresh*. https://innovation.cms.gov/strategic-direction-whitepaper

18. Medicaid and CHIP Payment and Access Commission. Federal medical assistance percentage. 2022. https://www.macpac.gov/subtopic/matching-rates/

19. Freed M, Damico A, Neuman T. Medicare advantage 2022 spotlight: first look. *Kaiser Family Foundation*. Published November 2, 2021. https://www.kff.org/medicare/issue-brief/ medicare-advantage-in-2022-enrollment-update-and-key-trends/

20. Terry K, Muhlestein D. Medicare advantage for all? Not so fast. *Health Affairs*. Published March 11, 2021. https://www.healthaffairs.org/do/10.1377/forefront.20210304.136304

21. Hinton E, Stolyar L. 10 things to know about Medicaid managed care. *Kaiser Family Foundation*. Published February 23, 2022. https://www.kff.org/medicaid/issue-brief/10-things-to-know-about-medicaid-managed-care/

22. Avalere. CMMI's financial impact on Medicare spending challenging to project (Updated). Published January 14, 2020. https://avalere.com/insights/cmmis-financial-impact-updated

23. Smith B. CMS innovation center at 10 years—progress and lessons learned. *N Engl J Med*. 2021;384(8):759-764. doi:10.1056/NEJMsb2031138

24. Ollove M. 3 states pursue public option for health coverage as feds balk. *PEW*. Published July 22, 2021. https://www.pewtrusts.org/en/research-and-analysis/blogs/stateline/ 2021/07/22/3-states-pursue-public-option-for-health-coverage-as-feds-balk

25. Carlton S, Kahn J, Lee M. Cascade select: insights from Washington's public option. *Health Affairs*. Published August 30, 2021. https://www.healthaffairs.org/do/10.1377/forefront .20210819.347789

26. Riotta C. GOP aims to kill Obamacare yet again after failing 70 times. *Newsweek*. Published August 29, 2022. https://www.newsweek.com/gop-health-care-bill-repeal-and-replace-70-failed-attempts-643832

27. Tolbert J, Orgera K, Damico A. Key facts about the uninsured population. *Kaiser Family Foundation*. Published November 6, 2020. https://www.kff.org/uninsured/issue-brief/ key-facts-about-the-uninsured-population/

28. Blumenthal D, Collins SR, Fowler EJ. The Affordable Care Act at 10 years—its coverage and access provisions. *N Engl J Med*. 2020;382(10):963-969. doi:10.1056/NEJMhpr1916091

29. Hall MA, McCue MJ. How has the Affordable Care Act affected health insurers' financial performance? *The Commonwealth Fund*. Published July 20, 2016. doi:10.26099/JNEK-Z932

30. Blumenthal D, Abrams MK. The Affordable Care Act at 10 years—payment and delivery system reforms. *N Engl J Med*. 2020;382(11):1057-1063. doi:10.1056/NEJMhpr1916092

31. Antos JR, Capretta JC. The ACA: Trillions? Yes. A Revolution? No. *Health Affairs*. Published April 10, 2020. https://www.healthaffairs.org/do/10.1377/forefront.20200406.93812/full/

32. Emanuel EJ. Name the much-criticized federal program that has saved the U.S. $2.3 trillion. Hint: it starts with affordable. *STAT*. Published March 22, 2019. https://www.statnews.com/2019/03/22/affordable-care-act-controls-costs/

33. Miller S, Altekruse S, Johnson N, Wherry LR. Medicaid and mortality: new evidence from linked survey and administrative data. NBER working paper no. 26081. National Bureau of Economic Research. 2019. https://www.nber.org/papers/w26081

34. Tikkanen R, Osborn R, Mossialos E, Djordjevic A, Wharton GA. International Health Care System Profiles: Canada. *The Commonwealth Fund*. Published June 5, 2020. https://www.commonwealthfund.org/international-health-policy-center/countries/canada

35. Tikkanen R, Osborn R, Mossialos E, Djordjevic A, Wharton GA. International health care system profiles: Germany. *The Commonwealth Fund*. Published June 5, 2020. https://www.commonwealthfund.org/international-health-policy-center/countries/germany#:~:text=About%2088%20percent%20of%20the,11%20percent%20through%20private%20insurance

36. Tikkanen R, Osborn R, Mossialos E, Djordjevic A, Wharton GA. International health care system profiles: Singapore. *The Commonwealth Fund*. Published June 5, 2020. https://www.commonwealthfund.org/international-health-policy-center/countries/singapore

37. Haskins J, Karnick ST. *The American Health Care Plan*. The Heartland Institute; 2021. https://www.heartland.org/_template-assets/documents/publications/AHCPa.pdf

38. Newport F. Americans' mixed views of healthcare and healthcare reform. *Gallup*. Published May 21, 2019. https://news.gallup.com/opinion/polling-matters/257711/americans-mixed-views-healthcare-healthcare-reform.aspx

39. Kliff S, Sanger-Katz M. Surprise medical bills cost Americans millions. Congress finally banned most of them. *The New York Times*. *TheUpshot*. Updated September 30, 2021. https://www.nytimes.com/2020/12/20/upshot/surprise-medical-bills-congress-ban.html

40. Cooper Z, Nguyen H, Shekita N, Morton FS. Out-of-network billing and negotiated payments for hospital-based physicians. *Health Aff (Millwood)*. 2020;39(1):24-32. doi:10.1377/hlthaff.2019.00507

41. CMS.gov. Surprise billing & protecting consumers. Published January 1, 2022. https://www.cms.gov/nosurprises/Ending-Surprise-Medical-Bills

42. Keith K. Doctors, air ambulance operators challenge interpretations of no surprises act. *Health Affairs*. Published December 6, 2021. https://www.healthaffairs.org/do/10.1377/forefront.20211206.44185/

43. Centers for Disease Control and Prevention. Opioids: prescription opioids. Accessed August 29, 2017. https://www.cdc.gov/opioids/basics/prescribed.html

44. Centers for Disease Control and Prevention. Prescribing practices: changes in opioid prescribing practices. Accessed August 13, 2019. https://www.cdc.gov/drugoverdose/deaths/prescription/practices.html

45. Centers for Disease Control and Prevention. Prescription opioid overdose death maps. Accessed June 6, 2022. https://www.cdc.gov/drugoverdose/deaths/prescription/maps.html

46. National Institute on Drug Abuse. Overdose death rates. Published January 20, 2022. https://www.drugabuse.gov/drug-topics/trends-statistics/overdose-death-rates

47. Appa A, Rodda LN, Cawley C, et al. Drug overdose deaths before and after Shelter-in-place orders during the COVID-19 pandemic in San Francisco. *JAMA Netw Open*. 2021;4(5):e2110452. doi:10.1001/jamanetworkopen.2021.10452

48. Hoffman J. Purdue Pharma is dissolved and Sacklers pay $4.5 billion to settle opioid claims. *The New York Times*. Published September 1, 2021. https://www.nytimes.com/2021/09/01/health/purdue-sacklers-opioids-settlement.html

49. National Conference of State Legislatures. Prescribing policies: states confront opioid overdose epidemic. Published June 30, 2019. https://www.ncsl.org/research/health/prescribing-policies-states-confront-opioid-overdose-epidemic.aspx

50. Mays JC, Newman A. Nation's first supervised drug-injection sites open in New York. *The New York Times*. November 2021. https://www.nytimes.com/2021/11/30/nyregion/supervised-injection-sites-nyc.html

51. Alzheimer's Association. 2022 Alzheimer's disease facts and figures. Special report: more than normal aging: understanding mild cognitive impairment. https://www.alz.org/media/Documents/alzheimers-facts-and-figures.pdf

52. Gandy S. 6 ways the FDA's approval of Aduhelm does more harm than good. *STAT*. Published June 15, 2021. https://www.statnews.com/2021/06/15/6-ways-fda-approval-aduhelm-does-more-harm-than-good/

53. The American Geriatrics Society. Food and Drug Administration's review of Biogen's drug Aducanumab for Alzheimer's disease. June 2, 2021. https://www.americangeriatrics.org/sites/default/files/inline-files/American%20Geriatrics%20Society_Letter%20to%20FDA%20Biogen%20Drug%20for%20Alzheimer%27s%20%28June%202021%29%20FINAL%20%281%29.pdf

54. Wehrwein P. 5 things you should know about the Aduhelm price cut. *Managed Healthcare Executive*. Published December 22, 2021. https://www.managedhealthcareexecutive.com/view/5-things-you-should-know-about-the-aduhelm-price-cut

55. Belluck P, Robbins R. Three F.D.A. Advisers resign over agency's approval of Alzheimer's drug. *The New York Times*. Updated September 2, 2021. https://www.nytimes.com/2021/06/10/health/aduhelm-fda-resign-alzheimers.html

56. Joseph A. Q&A: the CEO of the Alzheimer's Association on the approval of Aduhelm—and why critics should stop dwelling on the decision. *STAT*. Published June 16, 2021. https://www.statnews.com/2021/06/16/qa-ceo-alzheimers-association-on-aduhelm/

57. O'Brien S. Here's how one drug can be responsible for 50% of the hike in Medicare's Part B premiums. *CNBC*. Published December 12, 2021. https://www.cnbc.com/2021/12/12/why-one-drug-is-responsible-for-half-the-hike-medicare-part-b-premiums.html

7

Health Care Workforce

The health care workforce can seem overwhelming. If you walk into a hospital and start checking out work badges, you may end up being confused about who's who. What's a CNS (clinical nurse specialist)? Is a DO (doctor of osteopathic medicine) the same as an MD (doctor of medicine)? What does a licensed practical nurse (LPN) do? This chapter serves as a handy reference guide to the health care workforce—a summary of some important issues and a quick snapshot of the many important professions that make health care happen (Figure 7.1).

Professional Training

Education, Licensing, and Certification

Education

Educational requirements vary significantly for different health professions. Although some health care professionals receive all of their education on the

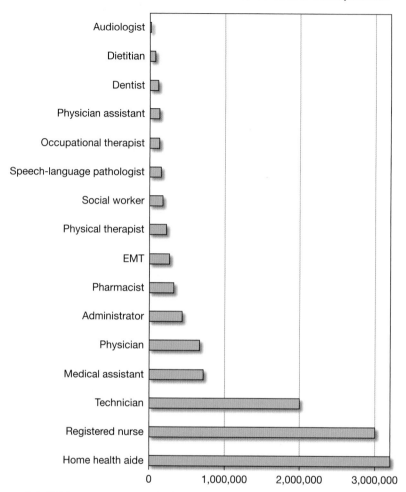

Number of U.S. Health Care Workers, Selected Occupations

Figure 7.1 EMT, emergency medical technician. (Adapted from Bureau of Labor Statistics, U.S. Department of Labor. *Occupational Outlook Handbook* (selected professions). Accessed December 2021. https://www.bls.gov/ooh/healthcare/home.htm)

job, the majority attend formal degree or certificate granting programs that may last anywhere from 9 months to 10 or more years. Some health care providers complete doctoral degrees that are specific to their profession. Upon graduation, members of particular professions—physicians, pharmacists, physician assistants or associates (PAs), podiatrists, and others—may enter postgraduate residency programs to receive additional training.

Licensing—Approval by the (State) Government

Licensing is legal approval from a state government to practice a profession. Not all health care roles require a license; for instance, many assistant and technician jobs do not. For those that do, licenses must be renewed every few years. Usually, renewal requires a fee and completion of continuing education in the field. Only those who are licensed are allowed to use certain titles associated with each profession.

The growth of national telemedicine providers has raised new questions about state licensing. Technically, a physician licensed in California, for example, cannot legally provide services to their patient who happens to be traveling to Missouri and wants a video visit, because this crosses state lines. Many such state-based restrictions were temporarily suspended during the pandemic, and some wonder if national licensing would make more sense.

Certification—Approval by a (National) Professional Organization

Board certification is a formal recognition of competence from a nongovernmental professional organization that is recognized across the country. Two types of certification are common. For professions that are licensed, certification allows workers to demonstrate competency in specific practice areas (eg, specialty physicians such as psychiatrists and cardiologists). For professions that aren't licensed, certification is a way of demonstrating quality to employers and the public. Some health care institutions require certification, even if the law does not. In some roles, such as with physicians, certification is the norm even if not technically required (Table 7.1).

Table 7.1 Examples of Professional Training in Health Care

	College	Formal training	Practical training	Specialized training	Licensing tests	Certification tests
Medical assistant	Optional	Optional certification programs, usually 1-2 years	On the job		None	Optional
Pharmacist	4 yr	PharmD, usually 4 yr	Optional 1- to 2-yr residency	On the job	Must pass two tests to get a state license	Optional but common in specialized work
General surgeon	4 yr	MD, usually 4 yr (can be combined with PhD for an extra ~3-5 yr)	5- to 7-yr residency	Optional fellowships lasting 1-3 yr	Must pass three tests to get a state license	Technically optional but uncommon not to become board certified

Graduate Medical Education

Physicians' degrees are awarded after completion of 4 years of medical school, but graduates must complete postgraduate residency training[a] in a medical specialty before they're allowed to practice medicine. Legally, physicians can gain their license after their intern (first) year of residency and can then begin practicing unsupervised, but this is a rare path. The default is to complete residency, during which these new physicians evaluate and treat patients under the supervision and guidance of more experienced attending physicians.

Residency programs are generally hospital based, and are governed by the Accreditation Council for Graduate Medical Education (ACGME). Residency lasts from 3 years (family medicine, pediatrics, internal medicine) to 7 years (neurosurgery), and training can be extended quite a bit longer with subspecialty fellowships.

Residents are technically not employees, and they lack the freedoms and protections that an employee might have.

First, they do not freely choose a residency position but are "matched" to one. The National Resident Matching Program uses an algorithm to match students with residencies based on mutual preference; those students who enter "the match" are contractually obligated to accept their given positions. However, the match is actually intended to serve as protection for applicants, easing and standardizing the previous, chaotic process of finding internships and residencies.

Second, resident salaries are fixed stipends—starting around $61,000 for an intern in 2021—and cannot be negotiated. This is despite the fact that residency programs get paid nearly $150,000 per resident by Medicare, and despite the fact that a fixed salary you are contractually obligated to take sounds a lot like price-fixing. A lawsuit in 2004 alleged just this—and in response, Congress simply decreed that antitrust law don't apply to graduate medical education.[1,2] However, we can get some idea of the financial value that residents provide to their institutions: In 2019, the University of New Mexico lost accreditation for their neurosurgery residency. To replace their 10 residents, they hired 23 nurse practitioners (NPs).[3]

Third, they work far more hours than is typical—compared both to other health care workers and to workers at large. Duty hours are capped at 80 hours per week, averaged over a 4-week period (meaning you can work 100 hours for 2 weeks as long as you "only" work 60 hours the next 2), and they cannot work longer than 28 hours in one shift. Although this pace can be brutally difficult, we should note that residents and physicians are far from

---

[a]Think *Scrubs* and *Grey's Anatomy* without the glamor.

the only workers used to insane hours, and it's not just well-paid investment bankers and lawyers—federal firefighters, for instance, often work 24-hour shifts, perform a role essential to their community, and make a starting salary often below $15 per hour.[4]

The upside to going through medical school and residency is that, once you finish, you are nearly guaranteed to get a job as an attending physician (contrast that to academia, for instance). Both medical school and residency slots have been limited by the federal government. There was a 25-year moratorium on medical school slots beginning in 1980, a misguided reaction to a fear that there would be too many physicians in the future. Residency slots, being funded by Medicare and Medicaid funds, have been capped since the Balanced Budget Act of 1997. Through this artificial shortage, physicians enjoy unusually good job—and wage—security.

Working Together

Scope of Practice and "Top of License"

In every state and for each licensed profession, laws regulate what each type of health care professional can and cannot do. This is termed the *scope of practice*. Ensuring that workers stick to their scope of practice is an important safety protection, to ensure that patients aren't being treated by someone who hasn't had adequate education and training. Even so, there is sometimes significant overlap in scope between professions. For instance, consider an LPN, a registered nurse (RN), and a physician working in a clinic. In this example, all three can administer vaccines, but only the RN and physician can assess medical complaints, and only the physician can diagnose disease and prescribe medication.

Scope of practice regulations can also differ significantly from state to state. For example, in New Mexico, NPs have full independent practice authority, can independently prescribe any medication that a physician can, and are recognized in state policy as primary care clinicians. In Georgia, NPs need a written protocol with a supervising physician to practice or prescribe medications, cannot prescribe certain controlled substances, and are not recognized in state policy as primary care clinicians.[5] As you can see, this gets complicated very quickly. Even beyond the state laws, you'll find further variation at the level of the health system, where privileges are determined by medical staffing committees and other groups.

Working at the "top of your license" means focusing on the most advanced tasks your training allows; that is, setting up a workflow such that, at the end of a patient clinic appointment, the LPN comes in to give a patient their vaccine, freeing the physician to move on to the next patient, all while the RN does phone triage to help decide who needs an urgent appointment that day. Although such workflows may be routine in the physical setting of a clinic, the breakdown of "who should do what" has needed to be reenvisioned for handling electronic health record (EHR) messages and population health–based interventions.

Sometimes licensing allows more freedom for a role, but they can't get reimbursed for it. There is probably no better example of this mismatch than for pharmacists. Pharmacists are highly trained and, in many states, can not only ensure the safe and accurate use of medications but also adjust those medications and educate patients to manage chronic disease. However, Medicare and Medicaid do not recognize pharmacists as "eligible providers" for billing (eligible providers are generally only clinicians), effectively disincentivizing pharmacists—or health systems that employ pharmacists—from working at the top of their license.[b]

In response to the COVID-19 pandemic, many states temporarily waived or relaxed the scope of practice laws to increase patient access, including waiving requirements for NPs and PAs to be supervised by a physician, and allowing pharmacists to independently administer vaccines and order COVID tests. Whether these changes will become permanent will vary by state, but it provided a natural experiment for changing the scope of practice regulations on access, outcomes, and cost.

Interprofessional Care Teams

Many models of health care delivery are organized around the concept of interprofessional, team-based medical care. Interprofessional care teams are composed of members from several different health professions who bring specialized knowledge, experience, and skills to the care of a given patient.

Interprofessional health care teams are particularly effective in caring for patients with multiple, complex medical and socioeconomic conditions. Let's consider the example of diabetes, which currently affects 13% of American adults.[6] Diabetes and its related conditions can affect nearly every organ system, and optimal care must be coordinated among several health care providers—the physician who diagnoses the condition and prescribes treatment, the nurse who helps the patient learn how to take medications and measure blood glucose properly, the physical therapist (PT) who works with activity limitations, the dietitian who guides the patient's eating regimen, and the podiatrist who treats the patient's foot ulcers and other complications.

---

[b]In 2021, a bill was introduced to fix this, the Pharmacy and Medically Underserved Area Enhancement Act, which would allow Medicare to reimburse pharmacists for Part B services that are already within their licensing scope of practice. https://www.pharmacist.com/APhA-Press-Releases/pharmacy-associations-applaud-introduction-of-bill-expanding-medicare-patients-access-to-pharmacist-services

Pharmacists assist in selecting the proper and affordable medication regimens, and social workers can help ensure that the patient can afford—and remain adherent with—the medications prescribed. Leveraging the knowledge and skills of each health care provider ensures that treatment is focused on the patient's needs and results in improved health outcomes.

Interprofessional teams have long been a part of medical care in settings such as hospital intensive care units (ICUs) and stroke care units. However, the team-based model has gradually been adopted in newer models of health care delivery embedded within population health systems (see Chapter 1). The hope is that interprofessional care teams will improve the coordination and delivery of patient care while mitigating health care costs. For example, alternative payment models (see Chapter 3) could provide a revenue stream that can support nonphysician team members through their potential impact on lowering health care spending (eg, many ACOs employ social workers to help patients free of charge, with the expectation that it will bring down total costs of care and therefore be worth the cost). New payment and incentive structures emphasize developing such teams, but effective adoption and implementation of team-based care still faces significant challenges.

As far back as 1972, the Institute of Medicine (IOM) recognized that changing medical care to a team-based model would involve wholesale changes at several levels: organizational, administrative, instructional, and national. In particular, the IOM noted that academic health centers would need to introduce a more collaborative educational model among the various health professions, particularly through integrating classroom instruction and clinical education.[8] Furthermore, systemic "macro-level" factors such as governmental policies, reimbursement, and regulation—not to mention societal and cultural values regarding medical care—introduce even more complexity to this issue. A transformation to team-based care faces significant barriers, which will require both collaboration and creativity to overcome.[7]

"Clinicians" and Scope of Practice

For thousands of years, physicians have been the dominant provider of medical services. Modern standards for their education and training were established in the 19th and early 20th centuries, forming the rigorous and lengthy process to becoming a physician that exists to this day.

Beginning in the 1960s, training programs for NPs and PAs, collectively known as advanced practice providers (APPs)[c], developed as a way to meet

---

[c]Previously known as mid-level providers or physician extenders.

the needs of an expanding population without access to enough physicians (Figure 7.2). The trade-off for shorter education programs and lack of residency training was restrictions on practice with requirements to work under the supervision of a physician.

Over time, APPs have greatly increased in number, and their scope of practice has expanded, as well. There are approximately 270,000 advanced practice nurses (APNs)[8] and approximately 130,000 PAs, and 35% of primary care practices employ at least one NP.[9] An increasing number of APPs practice in specialty care as well, including 75% of all PAs (Figure 7.3).[10] Nearly half of the states now permit NPs to practice without physician supervision, and NPs can apply for full admitting privileges at many hospitals. Similarly, a number of states permit nurse anesthetists to practice without physician supervision, especially those with large rural populations and physician shortages. For example, more than 80% of Kansas hospitals providing surgical services rely solely on nurse anesthetists rather than on physicians to provide anesthesia care. For their part, in 2021, a major PA organization rebranded as the American Academy of Physician *Associates*—eschewing the old term *assistants*.[11]

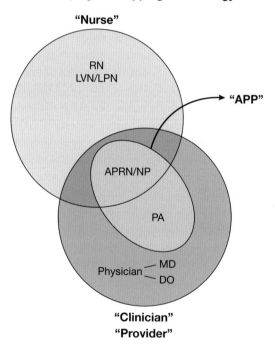

Clarifying Overlapping Terminology

"Nurse"

RN
LVN/LPN

"APP"

APRN/NP

PA

Physician — MD
— DO

"Clinician"
"Provider"

Figure 7.2 APP, advanced practice provider; APRN, advanced practice registered nurse; DO, doctor of osteopathic medicine; LPN, licensed practical nurse; LVN, licensed vocational nurse; MD, doctor of medicine; NP, nurse practitioner; PA, physician assistant; RN, registered nurse.

Expected Employment Growth 2020-2030

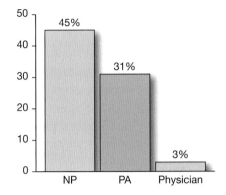

Figure 7.3 NP, nurse practitioner; PA, physician assistant. Information taken from the respective occupation pages from Bureau of Labor Statistics, U.S. Department of Labor. *Occupational Outlook Handbook*. Nurse anesthetists, nurse midwives, and nurse practitioners, physician assistants, and physicians and surgeons. Accessed April 19, 2022. https://www.bls.gov/ooh/healthcare/home.htm

Although physician education, training, and licensing are all highly standardized across the nation, APP education and training is much more variable, particularly for NPs. Some NPs have been nurses for decades before adding advanced training; others have entered accelerated programs that combine both nursing and NP training, going from no experience to full (and, in some cases, independent) practice in 3 years. Some NP programs are completed entirely online.[12] Further, although physicians must complete fellowships for specialized training such as cardiology and critical care, NPs have fewer restrictions and can switch from one field to another much more easily.

APPs' salaries are also lower than those of physicians, making them attractive to health care institutions.[d] As discussed in Chapter 3, physicians are increasingly employees rather than running their own practices. As such, some physicians view APPs not simply as partners in "extending" medical services but rather as competition.

This is the context for the current controversies over APP scope of practice reform. Emotions run high when discussing this topic because it involves perceived benefit or harm to patients, income, prestige, and professional identity. Although many physicians join APPs and APP organizations in championing partnership and growth, many other physicians and physician organizations oppose independent practice for APPs. They point to the more intensive training of physicians as evidence of their higher quality of care.

---

[d]APPs are reimbursed at 85% of the physician rate by Medicare. Physicians also receive extra compensation for supervising APPs.

The question is whether there is actually evidence of worse outcomes with decreased training. Some studies do investigate quality of care, cost of care, and patient preferences between APPs and physicians. The positive impact of NPs and PAs within the context of a physician-led team is well documented and sound.[13,14] The impact of their independent practice, however, is less easily studied. Given how important this issue is, research is surprisingly limited, and you can find studies to support whatever your point of view is.[e]

For anyone considering what scope of practice *should* be, it is important to consider the training that is necessary for the best health outcomes for the most patients while also considering the larger backdrop of politics, workforce development, and health care financing in which this debate takes place.

We should note, finally, the preference of patients. A 2018 study found that about half of patients choosing a new primary care clinician would choose a physician, a quarter would choose an APP, and a quarter don't have a preference. Those who opt for a physician prioritize qualifications, whereas those who opt for an APP prioritize bedside manner and convenience.[15]

Health Care Workforce Growth and Shortage: Wide-Ranging Implications

The health care industry is the #1 employer in the United States, employing more than one in eight of all American workers.[16] This workforce has grown over time, as our population has expanded and aged, and we anticipate even more growth in the future, adding an additional 11 million more jobs by 2030[17] (Figure 7.4).

Even as job growth accelerates, certain areas of the industry are experiencing a shortage of workers, especially as the COVID-19 pandemic influences what workers are willing to do—and for how much money. In particular, this shortage has been felt in the nursing field, ranging from assistants in nursing homes to highly trained specialty nurses in hospitals, and especially affecting rural areas. The American Hospital Association found that job vacancies for nurses and respiratory therapists increased by about 30% each from 2019 to 2020, and they estimate a total shortage of 3 million health care workers by 2026.[18]

What are the implications of this growth and shortage mismatch? Talking about labor issues may seem unglamorous, but the health care workforce—its size, composition, breakdown, and location—sits at the heart of so many issues discussed in this book. Here are just a few examples of how workforce issues play into topics you've read about in this book:

---

[e]If you'd like to read a point-counterpoint (from two physicians), see Suggested Reading.

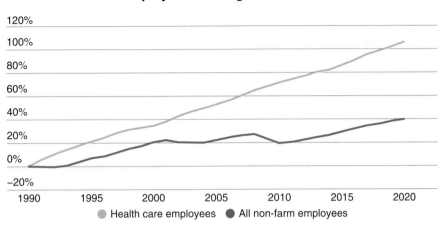

Figure 7.4 Adapted from The Center Square. Analysis: U.S. cities with the most health care workers. Lattice Publishing. Published June 3, 2020. https://www.the centersquare.com/national/analysis-u-s-cities-with-the-most-health-care-workers/article_ea3a1475-a825-5fa7-90c3-f575053b4372.html

- Health care delivery depends on the people doing the delivery. If we need more home-based care, then we need more home-based care workers— and the policy and reimbursement strategy to attract them. For instance, turnover in facilities such as nursing homes (already over 100% per year even before the pandemic[19]) likely reflect underpayment and poor working conditions, and the consequences of that turnover were felt keenly in the pandemic.
- Labor is the biggest expenditure for a hospital, and labor issues are at the forefront of a hospital chief operating officer (CEO)'s mind. Generally, health care workers' salaries are a major source of health care costs. Any time you talk about adding a program (or workers), you're increasing costs. And any time you talk about cutting costs, you're talking about cutting someone's job or salary.
- The fields of quality and digital health have added whole new arenas for health care workers. Thirty years ago, your hospital might have a handful of information technology (IT) guys; now they have dozens, if not hundreds, of EHR analysts, IT guys, and quality program administrators.

Even if you do not focus on labor in particular, as you consider any issue of delivery, reimbursement, or policy, it is always worth asking how the health care workforce might shape the issue—and how any potential solution might affect the workforce.

Workforce Diversity

American society is diverse, and so is the health care workforce. Yet, that diversity is not evenly spread throughout the health professions—and it is particularly skewed for positions of greater power, prestige, and income (Figure 7.5). For instance, women are half of the population and half of medical school graduates, whereas they only make up 5.5% of full clinical professors.[20] Hispanics are 18% of the workforce; yet they are significantly underrepresented in all diagnosing and treating jobs (such as nurse, PT, and physician) while overrepresented in assistant and technician jobs.[21]

Yet, evidence shows that patients often prefer to see health professionals who look like them, and may receive better communication and care when they do. In addition, research shows that female, Black, and Hispanic physicians are more likely to work with low-income patients in underserved areas.[22] Thus, workforce diversity may be another social determinant of health, and addressing it is important for patients as well as for workers.

In light of this, some call for public reporting and tracking of workforce diversity, as well as quality measures intended to incentivize it.[20,23]

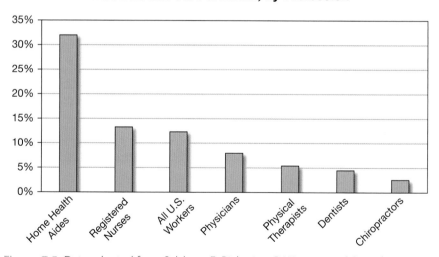

Black Health Care Workers, by Profession

Figure 7.5 Data adapted from Salsberg E, Richwine C, Westergaard S, et al. Estimation and comparison of current and future racial/ethnic representation in the US health care workforce. *JAMA Netw Open.* 2021;4(3):e213789. doi:10.1001/jamanetworkopen.2021.3789

Health Care Workforce Quick Reference Guide[24,25]

This is a quick guide to the health care professionals you're most likely to come across. Each profession includes the total number of persons in it, typical acronyms, gender (when available), what they do, how much they're paid, how they're educated, and more.

Assistant/Aide	NA/CNA/AA/CDA/PCT/Many More
Total number:	5.7 million
	Female: 85%; Male: 15%

Education:	Some nursing assistants/aides (NAs) receive no formal training and learn on the job, whereas others attend 1-year certificate/diploma programs or 2-year associate's degree programs.
Licensing:	State laws usually regulate scope of practice, but many states do not require a license for practice.
Average salary:	Varies depending on role. Lowest and highest paid: • NAs: Hourly: $15.41; annually: $32,050 • Occupational therapy assistants: Hourly: $30.49; annually: $63,420
Job description:	This category encompasses a wide variety of health care workers (excluding PAs and medical assistants) who are directed and supervised by licensed health care professionals. Aides are usually classified by the occupation of their supervisors: occupational therapy aides, anesthesia aides, and so on. These workers perform a wide range of vital tasks in all health care settings. Contact with patients can be extensive or quite minimal, depending on specific job requirements. The largest subtype of this professional, accounting for more than 40% of all aides and assistants, is NAs or patient care technicians (PCTs). NAs work under the supervision of RNs and practical nurses. They can perform many basic patient care duties, including helping patients eat, dress, and bathe; serving meals, making beds, and tidying up rooms; taking vital signs, helping patients ambulate, and escorting them to surgery or imaging. NAs are also the primary caregivers in most nursing homes.

Audiologist	AuD
Total number:	13,300
	Female: 83%; Male: 17%[26]

Education:	4-year doctoral degree program
Licensing:	Licensed in all 50 states
Average salary:	Hourly: $38.95; annually: $89,230
Job description:	Audiologists work with patients who have hearing, balance, or other ear problems such as tinnitus. They use a variety of tests to determine the severity and cause of hearing and balance disorders and determine treatments on their own or in conjunction with the patient's medical team. Audiologists often fit and program hearing aids, middle ear implants, and cochlear implants; examine and clean ear canals; and provide rehabilitative strategies for patients with hearing loss.

Health Care Chaplain/Hospital Chaplain	CC/BCC/CCC/BCCC
Total number:	8,030, with many more volunteers
Education:	At least 100 hours of didactic and 300 hours of clinical training in a health care setting
Licensing:	Not state licensed
Average salary:	Hourly: $27.68; annually: $57,580
Job description:	Health care chaplains are responsible for attending to the spiritual needs of patients, especially in hospitals, nursing homes, and hospice services. Seventy-five percent of hospitals employ them, and religiously affiliated hospitals are more likely than are secular hospitals to employ chaplains.[27] Chaplains may be trained clergy or lay people of any religion. Chaplains spend time one-on-one with patients, work with patients' families, provide spiritual support for medical staff, and may lead regular services in hospital chapels. Chaplains are often called on to provide bereavement support for patients and their families in the last hours of life.

Chiropractor	DC
Total number:	34,760 — Female: 24%; Male: 76%
Education:	4-year doctoral degree program
Licensing:	Licensed in all 50 states
Average salary:	Hourly: $40.30; annually: $83,830
Job description:	Chiropractors diagnose and treat patients with problems of the musculoskeletal system, especially back and neck pain. Many chiropractic treatments deal specifically with the spine, using manipulation of the spine as a primary intervention. Some chiropractors use additional procedures in their practices, including heat, water, light, massage, ultrasound, electric currents, and acupuncture. Chiropractors cannot prescribe drugs or perform major surgery.

Counselor	
Total number:	393,880 — Female: 70%; Male: 30%
Education:	Master's program in counseling, psychology, or social work
Licensing:	All states require at least a master's degree.

Counselor (*continued*)

Average salary:	Hourly: $24.78; annual: $51,550
Job description:	Counselors help individuals, families, or groups cope with physical, mental, and emotional disorders. Mental health counselors treat mental and emotional disorders and promote mental health. They are trained in a variety of therapeutic techniques to address issues such as depression, anxiety, substance addiction and abuse, suicidal impulses, stress, trauma, low self-esteem, and grief.

Dentist   DDS/DMD

Total number:	111,210 Female: 39% Male: 61%
Education:	4-year doctoral degree program. (Some oral and maxillofacial surgery specialists complete 6-year joint dentistry/general surgery residencies and receive both a DMD [Doctor of Medicine in Dentistry] and a DDS [Doctor of Dental Surgery] upon graduation.)
Licensing:	Licensed in all 50 states
Average salary:	Hourly: $89.57; annually: $186,300
Job description:	Dentists are the primary providers of tooth, gum, mouth, and masticatory system care in the United States. They are permitted to perform many of the duties of physicians, including taking histories, ordering and interpreting imaging, making diagnoses, prescribing medication, and performing surgery, but are restricted to the oral cavity and masticatory system. Additional qualifications or training are required to carry out complex treatments such as dental implants and oral and maxillofacial surgery. Some dentists, especially dental surgeons, have full hospital privileges, whereas most others have courtesy privileges or no hospital relationships.

Dietitian   RD/LD/LDN

Total number:	66,330 Female: 90% Male: 10%
Education:	A 3- to 4-year undergraduate degree program or a 1- to 2-year master's degree program
Licensing:	Laws vary by state. The title "Registered Dietitian" (RD) denotes graduation from an accredited dietetics program and passage of a national certification exam.

(*continued*)

Dietitian (*continued*) RD/LD/LDN

Average salary:	Hourly: $30.84; annually: $64,150
Job description:	Dietitians take detailed nutritional histories, assess metabolic and functional status, and work with other health professionals to develop appropriate diets for patients. This often involves designing diets to manage medical conditions such as diabetes or in response to treatments such as chemotherapy. Dietitians are also centrally involved in selecting the feeding method (ie, through an intravenous [IV] line) and composition of nutritional support for patients who cannot eat.

Emergency Medical Technician/Paramedic EMT

Total number:	257,700 (excluding volunteers) Female: 36%; Male: 64%
Education:	Training varies from around 100 hours for EMT-Basic to over 1,000 hours for paramedics
Licensing:	Licensed in all 50 states, and most require certification by either the National Registry of Emergency Medical Technicians or by state-specific programs.
Average salary:	Hourly: $19.41; annually: $40,370
Job description:	Emergency medical technicians (EMTs) and paramedics are responsible for quickly responding to emergency situations, assessing and stabilizing victims' medical conditions, and transporting victims to the nearest medical facility via ambulance or helicopter. Typical responsibilities also vary by training, as follows: • EMT-Basic: Noninvasive procedures such as bag-valve-mask ventilation, splinting, and automated external defibrillation • EMT-Intermediate: Starting IV lines, placing nasogastric tubes, and administering a limited number of medications, such as epinephrine and albuterol • EMT-Paramedic: Administering a greater number of medications orally or via IV, including antipsychotics and narcotics, interpreting electrocardiography (ECG) reports, endotracheal intubations, blood transfusions, and thoracic decompressions[40]

Health Care Administrator

Total number:	429,800
Education:	Education varies greatly; some attend 2- or 3-year master's programs in health administration (MHA), public health (MPH), business administration (MBA), or public administration (MPA).

Health Care Administrator (*continued*)

Licensing:	All states require licensing for nursing home administrators, whereas licensing is generally not required for other areas of health care administration.
Average salary:	Varies widely, from around $50,000 per year for mid-level managers at outpatient/group practices to over $10 million per year for CEOs of private insurance companies. 2020 Median pay: $104,280 a year or $50.13 an hour
Job description:	Health care administrators plan, direct, coordinate, and supervise the delivery of health care. These workers are either specialists in charge of specific clinical departments or generalists who manage entire facilities or systems. This broad category includes a wide range of workers, from CEOs of large health care networks to office managers at small group practices. Some health care providers, especially those in solo practice, also perform administrative duties, but most health care institutions are operated by full-time health administrators.

Home Health Aide/Personal Health Aide   HHA/PHA

Total number:	3.2 million Female: 87%; Male: 13%
Education:	No specific education is required; most employers and states do not require a high school diploma. Aides are usually trained on the job. Home health aides (HHAs) undertake 75 hours of training, including 16 hours of supervised practical experience and an examination.
Licensing:	Varies by state
Average salary:	Hourly: $13.49; annually: $28,060
Job description:	HHAs provide help to the disabled, chronically ill, elderly, cognitively impaired, and others who need assistance in their own homes or in residential facilities. They provide light housekeeping and homemaking tasks such as laundry, changing bed linens, shopping for food, and planning and preparing meals. The aides also may help clients get out of bed, bathe, dress, and groom. Some accompany clients to health-related appointments or on other errands.

Medical Assistant   MA/CMA/RMA/CCMA/NCMA

Total number:	710,200 Female: 91%; Male: 9%
Education:	Some receive no formal training and learn on the job, whereas others attend 1-year certificate/diploma programs or 2-year associate's degree programs.

(*continued*)

Medical Assistant (*continued*)	MA/CMA/RMA/CCMA/NCMA
Licensing:	No state requires licensing, but some require permits for certain procedures such as phlebotomies and injections. Voluntary certification programs and examinations are available from national organizations.
Average salary:	Hourly: $17.75; annually: $36,930
Job description:	Medical assistants perform administrative and clinical duties to keep offices running smoothly and to ensure patients are cared for. Specific tasks often include taking vital signs, preparing patients for examination, assisting with procedures and treatments, preparing and administering medications, collecting and processing patient specimens for medical tests, and scheduling appointments.

Medical Scientist		
Total number:	108,550	Female: 50%; Male: 50%
Education:	Although there are no specific educational requirements, most complete a 3- to 6-year doctoral degree program in an area of biological science.	
Licensing:	Although medical scientists are not licensed by any state, those who interact medically with patients or administer drugs must also be licensed clinicians (physician, nurse, etc).	
Average salary:	Hourly: $48.94; annually: $101,800	
Job description:	Medical scientists conduct biomedical research to advance knowledge of life processes and of other living organisms that affect human health, including viruses, bacteria, and other infectious agents. They also engage in laboratory research, clinical investigation, technical writing, drug development, regulatory review, and related activities. Many medical scientists divide their time between clinical practice and research activities.	

Nurse: The Many Types

Practical Nurse/Vocational Nurse		LPN/LVN
Total number:	676,440	Female: 91%; Male: 9%
Education:	A 12- to 18-month certificate program	
Licensing:	Licensed in all 50 states	
Average salary:	Hourly: $24.08; annually: $50,090	

Practical Nurse/Vocational Nurse (*continued*)   LPN/LVN

Job description: Practical nurses provide patient care under direction of an RN, a physician, or an APP. They perform many of the same duties as RNs but are not allowed to conduct comprehensive patient assessments or perform certain procedures and functions (specifics vary from state to state). For example, they may be allowed to remove catheters and IV lines but not place them. Major functions of LPNs in the hospital include administering medications, taking and recording vital signs, dressing wounds, feeding patients, performing ECGs, and assisting patients with dressing, hygiene, bathroom care, and walking. Many LPNs go on to become RNs at a later date.

Registered Nurse   RN

Total number: 2.99 million   Female: 87%;   Male: 13%

Education: Several educational paths are available to become an RN:
                    • Bachelor's degree (BSN): A 3- to 4-year university program
                    • Accelerated BSN: A 12- to 18-month program for students with non-nursing bachelor's degrees; leads to a BSN at a university or nursing college
                    • Associate's degree (ASN, AAS, ADN): A 2-year program at a community or junior college
                    • Master's entry level (MSN, MEPN): A 3- to 4-year graduate program for students with non-nursing bachelor's degrees
                    Completion of one of these paths allows a graduate nurse to take the national licensure exam.

Licensing: Licensed in all 50 states

Average salary: Hourly: $38.47; annually: $80,010

Job description: Nurses are the largest group of employees in the health care field, and they often spend more time with the patient and family members than does any other health care professional. RNs play a variety of roles in both inpatient and outpatient institutions, and their work responsibilities vary accordingly. Every new patient admitted to a hospital undergoes an initial nursing assessment by an RN to determine the patient's physical condition and functional status. During the course of a patient's stay, nurses conduct ongoing assessments, identify patient problems, maintain a plan of care, perform interventions, and evaluate the results of interventions within their scope of practice. Such independent interventions include symptom management, patient and family education, and skin and wound care. Other actions are specified by institutional protocol or in the "patient orders" that are submitted by physicians and other health care providers. Because nurses spend the most time with patients, they often confer with other members of the care team regarding the management of patients.

(continued)

| Registered Nurse (*continued*) | RN |

Hospital RNs are responsible for a broad range of patient care activities, including vital sign monitoring; starting, regulating, and maintaining IVs and catheters; delivering oxygen therapies, medication administration; obtaining blood and tissue specimens for laboratory testing; ambulating patients; educating patients and their family members; supervising and directing practical nurses and NAs; discharge planning and instruction; and charting and maintaining the medical record.

In most hospitals, nurses are assigned to a care team in a single location or medical unit. A "nurse manager" is the RN responsible for administration and supervision of that unit; another RN acts as a "charge nurse," supervising the other RNs and patients and conferring with the medical staff. All hospitals employ a chief nursing executive (title may differ by institution) to provide central nursing administration.

Advanced Practice Nurse

Advanced practice nurses (commonly referred to as APNs or advanced practice registered nurses [APRNs]) are RNs who have completed specialized graduate training in one of the four areas listed subsequently and have a broader scope of practice for diagnosis and treatment than do RNs. The United States has more than 270,000 practicing APRNs. All four types are licensed separately in all 50 states.

RNs who wish to become an APN must complete a master's program (MSN) or doctorate of nursing practice program (DNP). Programs are 2 to 4 years and require a BSN and an RN license for admission. Some, but not all, programs require clinical work experience as an RN in a related field before applying. Nursing research doctorate programs (DNS/DNSc) are also available, lasting 4 to 6 years, for nurses who would like to focus on research as a primary career.

APRN (Advanced Practice Registered Nurse) types

Nurse Practitioners (NP/CNP/CRNP) are permitted to perform most of the duties of physicians, such as taking histories, making diagnoses, prescribing medication and performing limited procedures. Average yearly salary is $114,510.

Clinical Nurse Midwives (CNM/CNMW/CM/NM/CPM) are providers of OB/GYN (obstetrician/gynecologist) services with an emphasis on pregnancy and childbirth. Their scope of practice is similar to that of NPs and PAs; they can diagnose and treat most conditions in the field of obstetrics. In roughly half of states, CNMs can practice and prescribe independently; in the others, they need to collaborate with a supervising physician.[28] Average yearly salary is $115,540.

Clinical Nurse Specialists (CNSs) have a similar education and scope of practice as NPs but with a focus, typically, on a single condition or specialty, such as oncology or critical care, for which they provide advanced nursing care. In addition to direct patient care, CNSs engage in teaching, mentoring, research, management, and systems improvement. CNSs are allowed to prescribe medications in some states.[29]

Nurse Anesthetists (CRNAs) specialize in administering sedation and anesthesia. Most states allow CRNAs to practice independently, whereas some require collaboration with a supervising physician. CRNAs are the primary provider of anesthesia in many rural locations. Average yearly salary is $189,190.

Occupational Therapist		OT/OTR/MOT/MSOT/OTD
Total number:	126,610	Female: 85%; Male: 15%
Education:	A 2.5- to 3.5-year master's or doctoral degree program	
Licensing:	Licensed in all 50 states	
Average salary:	Hourly: $42.06; annually: $87,480	
Job description:	Occupational therapists (OTs) help people with medical conditions and disabilities achieve greater function and independence in their lives by promoting meaningful activities or "occupations" such as dressing, cooking, eating, working, and going to school. Exercises may be used to increase strength and dexterity to restore function after illness or injury, whereas compensatory or alternative strategies may be taught for coping with permanent disabilities. For example, OTs select and teach the use of adaptive devices such as wheelchairs, orthoses, eating aids, and dressing aids. Hospital-based OTs are often centrally involved in the discharge planning process, recommending the appropriate level of care for the patient postdischarge—eg, nursing facility, rehab, home with assistance, and so on.	

Optometrist		OD
Total number:	36,690	Female: 46%; Male: 54%[30]
Education:	4-year doctoral degree program	
Licensing:	Licensed in all 50 states	
Average salary:	Hourly: $60.31; annually: $125,440	
Job description:	Optometrists are the primary providers of eye care in the United States. They are permitted to do many of the duties of physicians, including taking histories, ordering and interpreting imaging, and diagnosing conditions of the eye. Regulations on procedures and prescribing medications vary by state. Optometrists are commonly confused with other eye health professionals; to clarify, ophthalmologists are physicians who specialize in eye care, whereas optometrists make, fit, and help patients select eyeglasses and contacts.	

Pharmacist   PharmD/RPh

Total number:	315,470	Female: 58%; Male: 42%
Education:	4-year doctoral degree program. Many programs combine undergraduate and graduate work into a 6-year degree.	
Licensing:	Licensed in all 50 states	
Average salary:	Hourly: $60.32; annually: $125,460	
Job description:	Pharmacists are responsible for receiving prescriptions and preparing medicines for patients. They are also legally responsible for educating patients about medications, and they work with physicians to optimize pharmacotherapy, for example, by reducing dangerous drug interactions and side effects. They are integral parts of the care team particularly in hospitals. In many states, pharmacists enter into "collaborative practice agreements" with physicians, which may enable them to modify medication regimens and prescribe a limited number of drugs. Pharmacists can administer medications and immunizations, although this varies from state to state. Pharmacists' scope of practice is much greater in federal settings such as the VA.	

Physical Therapist   PT/DPT/MPT/MSPT/BSPT

Total number:	220,870	Female: 67%; Male: 33%
Education:	3-year doctoral degree program	
Licensing:	Licensed in all 50 states	
Average salary:	Hourly: $44.08; annually: $91,680	
Job description:	PTs diagnose and treat movement-related conditions that limit strength, balance, coordination, flexibility, and functional independence. PTs may use therapeutic exercises, stretching, range-of-motion exercises and mobilization, functional training, manual therapy, use of assistive and adaptive devices/equipment to enhance function, and therapeutic modalities and electrical stimulation to manage pain. They often recommend long-term exercise plans for patients to complete on their own following treatment. Hospital-based PTs are often centrally involved in the discharge planning process, recommending the appropriate level of care for the patient postdischarge—for example, nursing facility, rehab, home with assistance, and so on.	

Physician	**MD (Allopathic)/DO (Osteopathic)**
Total number:	663,060 Female: 41%; Male: 59%
Education:	4-year doctoral degree program and required postgraduate residency of 3 to 7 years
Licensing:	Licensed in all 50 states
Average salary:	Varies depending on specialty, examples include the following:
• General pediatrician:	• Hourly: $95.40; annually: $198,420
• Psychiatrist:	• Hourly: $120.08; annually: $249,760
• Orthopedic surgeon:	• Hourly $147.22; annually: $306,220
Job description:	Physicians diagnose and treat injury and disease and are the primary educators and advisers of patients. Physicians examine patients, obtain medical histories, and order, perform, and interpret diagnostic tests. They prescribe medications and perform surgeries and other procedures. Specialties include anesthesiology, family medicine, internal medicine, pediatrics, obstetrics and gynecology, psychiatry, and surgery, as well as many subspecialties. Although only one-fifth of health expenditures go directly to physician services (and only 8% to physician salaries[31]), their clinical decisions determine up to 90% of total health expenditures (https://pubmed.ncbi.nlm.nih.gov/12409848/). Osteopathic physicians have a virtually identical training and scope of practice as allopathic physicians.

Physician Assistant (or Associate)	**PA/PA-C**
Total number:	125,280 Female: 64%; Male: 36%
Education:	3-year master's degree program
Licensing:	Licensed in all 50 states
Average salary:	Hourly: $55.81; annually: $116,080
Job description:	Despite the misleading name, PAs are clinicians who are permitted to perform most of the duties of a physician, such as taking histories, making diagnoses, prescribing medication, and performing limited procedures, but they must do so under physician supervision or collaboration. Surgical PAs assist surgeons during procedures and suture wounds but do not perform surgery themselves. PAs are allowed to prescribe medications in all 50 states, but some states restrict the prescription of controlled substances.

Podiatrist		**DPM**
Total number:	9,710	Female: 27%; Male: 73%[32]
Education:	4-year doctoral degree program, followed by a required 3-year residency	
Licensing:	Licensed in all 50 states	
Average salary:	Hourly: $72.65; annually: $151,110	
Job description:	Podiatrists are the primary providers of foot and ankle care in the United States.[33] They are permitted to perform many of the duties of physicians, including taking histories, ordering and interpreting imaging, making diagnosis, prescribing medication, and performing surgery, but their work is restricted to the foot and ankle. Hospital relationships vary by institution; some podiatrists are granted full hospital admitting privileges, and some coadmit with physicians.	

Clinical Psychologist		**CP/LCP/LP/PsyD**
Total number:	111,320	Female: 53%; Male: 47%[34]
Education:	A 4- to 5-year doctoral degree program, followed by a required 1-year clinical internship	
Licensing:	Licensed in all 50 states	
Average salary:	Hourly: $42.93; annually: $89,290	
Job description:	Clinical psychologists are mental health providers who focus on the mind and behavior. They assess and diagnose mental illnesses such as mood, anxiety, behavior, and adjustment disorders, and treat these conditions through interactive therapy. Common interventions include cognitive restructuring, behavioral management strategies, motivational interviewing, and modifying family patterns of interaction. Health psychologists are a specialty of clinical psychologists who often work in health care settings. Their activities include identifying strategies to promote adherence and increase coping, making behavioral changes to support physical and emotional health, and helping with pain management.	

Social Worker		**LSW/LICSW/LCSW/CSW/LCS/LMSW**
Total number:	176,110	Female: 73%; Male: 27%
Education:	A 3- to 4-year undergraduate degree program or 2-year master's degree program	

Social Worker (*continued*)   LSW/LICSW/LCSW/CSW/LCS/LMSW

Licensing:	Many states offer a tiered system of social work licenses based on education and clinical experience (eg, social worker, clinical social worker, and independent clinical social worker).
Average salary:	Hourly: $29.07; annually: $60,470
Job description:	Social workers in hospitals and other medical settings are often responsible for helping patients with nonmedical issues that affect their health. For example, many hospital-based social workers make discharge plans for patients to ensure that they will go to a safe place to recuperate upon leaving the hospital. This may include finding shelter for homeless patients, arranging home health care services, transferring patients to rehabilitation centers, and planning for follow-up visits at the hospital or clinic. Social workers often help low-income patients apply for health insurance and financial support and manage advance directives, patient support groups, and patient transportation. Social workers are found in a number of other health care roles outside the hospital, including therapist; in fact, the nation's largest group of mental health service providers are clinical social workers working as therapists.[35]

Speech-Language Pathologist   SLP

Total number:	148,450 Female: 94%; Male: 6%
Education:	A 2- to 3-year master's degree program, followed by a required 36-week clinical fellowship
Licensing:	Licensed in all 50 states
Average salary:	Hourly: $40.02; annually: $83,240
Job description:	Speech-language pathologists (SLPs) work with patients who have impairments in speaking, producing, or comprehending language, and with cognition and swallowing that result from congenital or acquired disease, syndrome, or injury. SLPs help patients develop or recover functional communication and swallowing skills. For individuals with little or no speech capability, SLPs may select augmentative or alternative communication methods, including automated devices and sign language, and teach their use.

Technician/Technologist	XT/RDMS/CPhT/NMT/CVT/More	
Total number:	2 million	Female: 71%; Male: 29%
Education:	Many technicians receive no formal training and learn on the job. Others attend 6-month to 1-year certificate/diploma programs, 2-year associate's degree programs, or 4-year bachelor's degree programs.	
Licensing:	Many states do not require licensing. Voluntary certification is offered by several national organizations.	
Average salary:	Varies depending on role. Lowest and highest paid: • Dietetic technicians: Hourly: $15.83; annually: $32,920 • Nuclear medicine technicians: Hourly: $39.46; annually: $82,080	
Job description:	This category encompasses a wide variety of health care workers (excluding EMTs) who deal primarily with specialized medical equipment. Examples include sonographers, who operate ultrasounds; pharmacy technicians, who prepare medicines; and radiology technologists, who operate imaging equipment such as computed tomography (CT) or magnetic resonance imaging (MRI) scanners. Generally, a health care professional such as a physician will order a test or treatment for a patient; technicians and technologists are then responsible for using their equipment to complete the order in a timely and accurate manner. Technicians and technologists work under the broad supervision of a physician but most of their day-to-day activities are performed independently.	

References

1. Weinmeyer R. Challenging the medical residency matching system through antitrust litigation. *AMA J Ethics.* 2015;17(2):147-151. doi:10.1001/virtualmentor.2015.17.2.hlaw1-1502

2. Carmody B. The match, part 5: the lawsuit. *The Sheriff of Sodium.* Published March 3, 2021. Accessed April 24, 2022. https://thesheriffofsodium.com/2021/03/03/the-match-part-5-the-lawsuit/

3. Boetel R. Residents complained before loss of accreditation, UNM says. *Albuquerque Journal.* Published December 15, 2019. https://www.abqjournal.com/1401413/residents-complained-before-loss-of-accreditation-unm-says.html

4. Ogrysco N. Interior, USDA to implement pay raises for federal firefighters later this month. *Federal News Network.* Accessed April 24, 2022. https://federalnewsnetwork.com/pay/2021/08/interior-usda-to-implement-pay-raises-for-federal-firefighters-later-this-month/

5. Scope of Practice Policy. Nurse practitioners overview Accessed April 24, 2022. https://scopeofpracticepolicy.org/practitioners/nurse-practitioners/

6. National Diabetes Statistics Report 2020: estimates of diabetes and its burden in the United States. Accessed April 24, 2022. https://www.cdc.gov/diabetes/pdfs/data/statistics/national-diabetes-statistics-report.pdf

7. Interprofessional Education Collaborative Expert Panel. Core competencies for interprofessional collaborative practice. https://www.aacom.org/docs/default-source/insideome/ccrpt05-10-11.pdf

8. Bureau of Labor Statistics, U.S. Department of Labor, Nurse anesthetists, nurse midwives, and nurse practitioners. *Occupational Outlook Handbook*. Accessed April 19, 2022. https://www.bls.gov/ooh/healthcare/nurse-anesthetists-nurse-midwives-and-nurse-practitioners.htm

9. Martsolf GR, Barnes H, Richards MR, Ray KN, Brom HM, McHugh MD. Employment of advanced practice clinicians in physician practices. *JAMA Intern Med.* 2018;178(7):988-990. doi:10.1001/jamainternmed.2018.1515

10. National Commission on Certification of Physician Assistants. 2020 statistical profile of certified physician assistants by specialty. Annual report. https://www.nccpa.net/wp-content/uploads/2021/12/2020-Specialty-report-Final.pdf

11. AAPA. Title change. June-July, 2021. https://www.aapa.org/title-change/#tci-implementation

12. Auerbach DI, Buerhaus PI, Staiger DO. Implications of the rapid growth of the nurse practitioner workforce in the US. *Health Aff (Millwood).* 2020;39(2):273-279. doi:10.1377/hlthaff.2019.00686

13. Everett C, Thorpe C, Palta M, Carayon P, Bartels C, Smith MA. Physician assistants and nurse practitioners perform effective roles on teams caring for Medicare patients with diabetes. *Health Aff (Millwood).* 2013;32(11):1942-1948. doi:10.1377/hlthaff.2013.0506

14. Kleinpell RM, Grabenkort WR, Kapu AN, Constantine R, Sicoutris C. Nurse practitioners and physician assistants in acute and critical care: a concise review of the literature and data 2008-2018. *Crit Care Med.* 2019;47(10):1442-1449. doi:10.1097/CCM.0000000000003925

15. Leach B, Gradison M, Morgan P, Everett C, Dill MJ, Oliveira JS. Patient preference in primary care provider type. *Healthcare.* 2018;6(1):13-16. doi:10.1016/j.hjdsi.2017.01.001

16. Dowell EKP. Census Bureau's 2018 county business patterns provides data on over 1,200 industries. *United States Census Bureau*. Published October 14, 2020. https://www.census.gov/library/stories/2020/10/health-care-still-largest-united-states-employer.html

17. U.S. Bureau of Labor Statistics. Employment projections: 2020-2030 summary. Published September 8, 2021. https://www.bls.gov/news.release/ecopro.nr0.htm

18. American Hospital Association. Fact Sheet: strengthening the health care workforce. Published June 2020. https://www.aha.org/fact-sheets/2021-05-26-fact-sheet-strengthening-health-care-workforce

19. Gandhi A, Yu H, Grabowski DC. High nursing staff turnover in nursing homes offers important quality information. *Health Aff (Millwood).* 2021;40(3):384-391. doi:10.1377/hlthaff.2020.00957

20. Rotenstein LS, Reede JY, Jena AB. Addressing workforce diversity—a quality-improvement framework. *N Engl J Med.* 2021;384(12):1083-1086. doi:10.1056/NEJMp2032224

21. U.S. Department of Health and Human Services, Health Resources and Services Administration, National Center for Health Workforce Analysis. Sex, race, and ethnic diversity of U.S, health occupations (2011-2015). 2017. https://bhw.hrsa.gov/sites/default/files/bureau-health-workforce/data-research/diversity-us-health-occupations.pdf

22. Health Professionals for Diversity Coalition. Fact Sheet: the need for diversity in the health care workforce. *AAPCHO*. https://www.aapcho.org/wp/wp-content/uploads/2012/11/NeedForDiversityHealthCareWorkforce.pdf

23. Salsberg E, Richwine C, Westergaard S, et al. Estimation and comparison of current and future racial/ethnic representation in the US Health Care Workforce. *JAMA Netw Open*. 2021;4(3):e213789. doi:10.1001/jamanetworkopen.2021.3789

24. Bureau of Labor Statistics, U.S. Department of Labor. *Occupational Outlook Handbook*. Accessed December 2021. https://www.bls.gov/ooh/healthcare/home.htm

25. Bureau of Labor Statistics, U.S. Department of Labor. Labor force statistics from the current population health survey. Accessed December 2021. https://www.bls.gov/cps/cpsaat11.htm

26. Data USA. Audiologists. https://datausa.io/profile/soc/audiologists#about

27. Handzo G, Flannelly KJ, Hughes BP. Hospital characteristics affecting healthcare chaplaincy and the provision of chaplaincy care in the United States: 2004 vs. 2016. *J Pastoral Care Counsel*. 2017;71(3):156-162. doi:10.1177/1542305017720122

28. NCSBN. CNM Independent Practice Map. Updated September 8, 2021. https://www.ncsbn.org/5405.htm

29. NCSBN. CNM Independent Prescribing Map. Updated September 8, 2021. https://www.ncsbn.org/5410.htm

30. Data USA. Optometrists. https://datausa.io/profile/soc/optometrists

31. NPR. Are Doctors overpaid. Published March 12, 2019. https://www.npr.org/sections/money/2019/03/12/702500408/are-doctors-overpaid

32. Data USA. Podiatrists. https://datausa.io/profile/soc/podiatrists

33. Illinois Podiatric Medical Association. Job description. https://www.ipma.net/podiatric-medicine

34. Willyard C. Men: a growing minority? *American Psychological Association*. https://www.apa.org/gradpsych/2011/01/cover-men

35. American Board of Clinical Social Work. What is clinical social work? https://www.abcsw.org/what-is-clinical-social-work

We separated this book into chapters, but you may have noticed the tons of cross-referencing we did between sections. The reality is that many topics in health care fall under more than one heading. Let's synthesize some of what you've learned in this book by looking at the Hospital Readmissions Reduction Program (HRRP), a policy that, through a reimbursement disincentive, changed delivery.

Background

From Chapters 1, 3, and 6 of this book, you know that Medicare has long been concerned with reining in hospital spending. In the early 2000s, health service researchers began to highlight hospital *re*admissions—that is, patients who get admitted to the hospital again, less than 30 days after being discharged the first time—as a potential approach to lower costs while improving quality. From a financial perspective, the concern was that nearly 20% of all Medicare patients discharged from the hospital were readmitted within 30 days—adding up to 3.3 million rehospitalized Medicare patients and costing Medicare $26 billion annually.[1,2] From a quality perspective, the concern was that those high readmission rates were due to poor-quality inpatient care, or to patients being discharged too quickly without sufficient planning for the transition to home and outpatient care. Rather than paying extra for the work of good discharge planning and coordination—something many felt hospitals had the responsibility to be doing already—Medicare chose to penalize hospitals for having too many readmissions. The idea was that the threat of losing money would incentivize hospitals to invest in better discharge planning and transitions programs.

The Policy

HRRP was enacted as part of the ACA in 2012. HRRP focuses on initial admissions for certain conditions, shown in the following. The program started with three conditions and eventually expanded to six.

- Acute myocardial infarction ("heart attack")
- Heart failure
- Pneumonia
- Coronary artery bypass graft ("CABG" or bypass surgery)
- Chronic obstructive pulmonary disease (COPD)
- Hip and knee replacements

Starting with the patients admitted to the hospital for these conditions in a given 3-year time period, Medicare then calculates each hospital's readmission ratios for these conditions.

1. Count any unplanned readmission within 30 days after discharge (for any reason, not just the initial condition).
2. Risk-adjust for some factors (age, ICD-10 codes for medical comorbidities).
3. Compare the individual hospital's readmission rate to the average of all hospitals, as a ratio. (That is, if the hospital's admission rate was exactly equal to the average, the ratio would be 1.) Any ratio higher than 1 is considered evidence of "excess readmissions."

The ratio is used to determine penalties. The higher the ratio, the more the hospital gets penalized. Penalties are based on the amount the CMS reimburses annually for Medicare patient admissions, and hospitals cannot be penalized more than 3% of their Medicare reimbursement rate. This ranges into millions of dollars.[3] Some hospitals are exempt from penalties, such as critical access, children's, and psychiatric hospitals.

Delivery Change

Many hospitals invested significant resources into discharge planning, medication reconciliation, patient educators, and transitional care programs. This meant hiring new staff, setting up new electronic risk assessment and tracking systems, addressing patients' social needs (like transportation), and setting up postdischarge phone call or home visit programs.[1,4,5] Hospital systems can most easily coordinate care if they are part of a vertically integrated network (ie, hospital network that also owns clinics, sharing an EHR between clinicians and teams), whereas establishing communication systems between unconnected organizations takes extra work.[5]

The Results

Readmission rates decreased for all six conditions, although this leveled off after 2014 (Figure C.1). Risk-adjusted rates decreased significantly more than raw rates did; some researchers found this discrepancy to be due to the more intensive coding of diagnoses—with one study finding approximately 60% of the improvement in readmission rates was due to coding alone[6]— whereas some felt that there was also a true change in patient complexity.[7] Interestingly, throughout this time, *initial* admission rates for these conditions also fell, indicating that perhaps simpler cases were being managed in the outpatient setting, so a more complex mix of patients was getting admitted in the first place.[7]

There are a few elements of the HRRP's design that are worth noting. First, HRRP defines only inpatient hospitalizations—not observation stays or ED visits—as readmissions. Many hospitals have focused on changing patients from inpatient to observation status as a strategy to reduce HRRP penalties. Although readmission rates have decreased for targeted conditions, rates of observation stays and ED visits after inpatient stays have increased; as a result, the proportion of patients who return to a hospital within 30 days after discharge has not changed nearly as much as it would appear by looking at readmissions alone.[8] Furthermore, because of the statistical methods used by CMS, researchers estimate that up to a third of hospitals had readmissions measured (and potentially penalized) incorrectly by CMS.[9]

Second, it's possible that hospitals could get dinged for keeping more patients alive. This is because readmission ratios do not account for deaths, and in theory hospitals that keep more patients alive are discharging a sicker

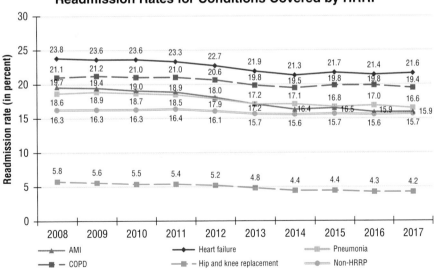

Figure C.1 AMI, acute myocardial infarction; COPD, chronic obstructive pulmonary disease; HRRP, Hospital Readmissions Reduction Program. (Adapted from MedPAC. Update: MedPAC's evaluation of Medicare's Hospital Readmission Reduction Program. Published December 2, 2019. https://www.medpac.gov/update-medpac-s-evaluation-of-medicare-s-hospital-readmission-reduction-program/)

group of people who are more prone to be readmitted.[8] Penalties for high *readmission* rates under the HRRP were up to 15 times higher than penalties for high *mortality* under a related CMS payment program.[10]

The actual effect of HRRP on mortality is somewhat less clear. Risk-adjusted mortality declined[7] (a trend beginning before HRRP was enacted), but several studies showed an increase in raw mortality for some conditions in some years, particularly for heart failure.[8] Overall, it's unclear whether any mortality increase was real, and whether HRRP had anything to do with it if so.

In the first 10 years of the program, 93% of the hospitals subject to HRRP were penalized at least once, and over 1,200 hospitals have been penalized every year.[11] Less than 2% of hospitals paid the maximum penalty,[1] but those penalties add up: in 2021 alone, over $500 million in penalties were paid to Medicare.[11]

Teaching hospitals, rural hospitals, and those that serve higher proportions of low-income beneficiaries were most likely to receive penalties,[a] and those with the smallest number of low-income beneficiaries were least likely to receive penalties. Because of this variation based on hospital characteristics, the 21st Century Cures Act updated HRRP to now compare hospitals within five peer groups based on each hospital's poverty rate rather than comparing all hospitals to the national average.[1,12]

Questions for Thought and Discussion

1. Risk adjustment is prevalent throughout value-based payment programs, driving a focus on maximizing coding of certain medical conditions. Notably, current risk adjustment programs do not account for social isolation, frailty, literacy, or income. What might an ideal risk adjustment process look like, being fair to providers that serve complex patient populations without incentivizing too much focus on coding?

2. Some aspects of the HRRP metric seem unfair, like comparing a safety net hospital to one in a wealthy area. Other aspects may hide worse quality, like the fact that people who die at home don't get counted as a readmission. How do you design a quality metric that gets at the outcome you want and can't be gamed? Is a more complex calculation always better, or are there times when a simple metric is better?

3. Medicare expects hospitals to coordinate a smooth transition home, but notably Medicare will not pay for home care items such as blood pressure monitors, medication management systems, or home care attendants. When it comes to safe discharge and delivering care at home, what is the provider's responsibility, and what is the payer's responsibility?

---

[a]Penalties did not include any risk adjustment for social determinants of health factors.

4. There is evidence that working within a hospital network or vertically integrated system makes communication and coordination around discharge much easier. Given this, how should we think about hospital network consolidation and its impact on quality? If much of the benefit is just from sharing the same EHR, then will interoperability achieve the same level of cooperation among different organizations? Are there other ways policy can encourage cooperation and coordination between different providers and organizations without market consolidation?

5. We require a high level of evidence to show that medications and devices will be effective and won't cause harm before they are approved and sold to consumers. Should policy be subjected to the same level of testing and rigor before it is implemented on a large scale?

6. Discharge and transitional care programs increase the workforce for patient educator, social worker, nursing, and administrator roles. Expanding medical teams to include nonclinician roles is a major strategy of population health and delivery innovations. At the same time, we know that health care worker wages drive a lot of spending. What is good about this expansion of the health care workforce? What is bad about it?

7. APMs and value-based payment try to align incentives to improve quality while lowering spending. Does it make sense in all cases to expect higher quality at lower costs? When should we expect to instead pay *more* for better care?

8. An important aspect in determining the success of a policy is understanding its goals. What were the HRRP's goals, and was HRRP a success?

References

1. NEJM Catalyst. Hospital Readmissions Reduction Program (HRRP). Published April 26, 2018. https://catalyst.nejm.org/doi/full/10.1056/CAT.18.0194

2. Agency for Healthcare Research and Quality. Conditions with the largest number of adult hospital readmissions by payer, 2011. Statistical Brief #172. Published April 2014. https://www.hcup-us.ahrq.gov/reports/statbriefs/sb172-Conditions-Readmissions-Payer.pdf

3. McIlvennan CK, Eapen ZJ, Allen LA. Hospital readmissions reduction program. *Circulation*. 2015;131(20):1796-1803. doi:10.1161/CIRCULATIONAHA.114.010270

4. Mays G, Li J, Clouser JM, et al. Understanding the groups of care transition strategies used by U.S. hospitals: an application of factor analytic and latent class methods. *BMC Med Res Methodol*. 2021;21:228. doi:10.1186/s12874-021-01422-7

5. Silow-Carroll S, Edwards JN, Lashbrook A. Reducing hospital readmissions: lessons from top-performing hospitals. *The Commonwealth Fund*. Published April 6, 2011. https://www.commonwealthfund.org/publications/case-study/2011/apr/reducing-hospital-readmissions-lessons-top-performing-hospitals

6. Ibrahim AM, Dimick JB, Sinha SS, Hollingsworth JM, Nuliyalu U, Ryan AM. Association of coded severity with readmission reduction after the hospital readmissions reduction program. *JAMA Intern Med*. 2018;178(2):290-292. doi:10.1001/jamainternmed.2017.6148

7. MedPAC. Update: MedPAC's evaluation of Medicare's Hospital Readmission Reduction Program. Published December 2, 2019. https://www.medpac.gov/update-medpac-s-evaluation-of-medicare-s-hospital-readmission-reduction-program/

8. Wadhera RK, Yeh RW, Joynt Maddox KE. The Hospital Readmissions Reduction Program—time for a reboot. *N Engl J Med*. 2019;380(24):2289-2291. doi:10.1056/NEJMp1901225

9. Shen C, Wadhera RK, Yeh RW. Misclassification of hospital performance under the Hospital Readmissions Reduction Program: implications for value-based programs. *JAMA Cardiol*. 2021;6(3):332-335. doi:10.1001/jamacardio.2020.4746

10. Gupta A, Fonarow GC. The Hospital Readmissions Reduction Program-learning from failure of a healthcare policy. *Eur J Heart Fail*. 2018;20(8):1169-1174. doi:10.1002/ejhf.1212

11. Rau J. 10 Years of Hospital Readmissions Penalties. Published November 4, 2021. https://www.kff.org/health-reform/slide/10-years-of-hospital-readmissions-penalties/

12. Boccuti C, Casillas G. Aiming for fewer hospital u-turns: the Medicare Hospital Readmission Reduction Program. https://www.kff.org/medicare/issue-brief/aiming-for-fewer-hospital-u-turns-the-medicare-hospital-readmission-reduction-program/

Data treasure trove	**Kaiser Family Foundation:** https://www.kff.org/
	Commonwealth Fund: https://www.commonwealthfund.org/
	RAND Corporation: https://www.rand.org/topics/health-health-care-and-aging.html
	Health Affairs: https://www.healthaffairs.org/
	MedPAC reports: https://www.medpac.gov/#
	MACPAC reports: https://www.macpac.gov/topics/
Keeping up with news	**Health Affairs**—Forefront (blog), sign up for their email newsletter, listen to their podcasts. https://www.healthaffairs.org/forefront
	STAT—news, podcasts. https://www.statnews.com/
	The Incidental Economist—a great, multifaceted blog. https://theincidentaleconomist.com/wordpress/
Books	*The Social Transformation of American Medicine* by Paul Starr
	An American Sickness by Elisabeth Rosenthal
	Priced Out by Uwe Reinhardt
	Bottle of Lies by Katherine Eban
	Health Care Advocacy by Laura Sessums, et al.
	Why Are the Prices So Damn High? by Alex Tabarrok and Eric Helland
	Understanding Patient Safety by Bob Wachter and Kiran Gupta
	The Ten Year War by Jonathan Cohn
	The Digital Doctor by Bob Wachter
	The Checklist Manifesto by Atul Gawande
	The Immortal Life of Henrietta Lacks by Rebecca Skloot
	Deep Medicine by Eric Topol
	Health Care Reform: What It Is, Why It's Necessary, How It Works by Jonathan Gruber
Particular topics	**The ACO Show Podcast**—about alternative payment models and value-based care. https://resources.aledade.com/aco-show-podcasts
	MedPAC Payment Basics—explainers on all aspects of Medicare payment. https://www.medpac.gov/document-type/payment-basic/
	Institute of Healthcare Improvement Courses—learn about quality improvement basics. http://www.ihi.org/education/IHIOpenSchool/Pages/default.aspx
	Drugchannels.net—blog and reports about pharmaceutical economics and the drug distribution system. http://drugchannels.net/

Retraction Watch—database for retracted studies. https://retractionwatch.com/

Health Care Triage—videos about health policy, economics, and delivery topics. https://www.youtube.com/channel/UCabaQPYxxKepWUsEVQMT4Kw

Commonwealth Fund International Comparative Profiles: https://www.commonwealthfund.org/international-health-policy-center/system-profiles

Oregon Medicaid Experiment: https://www.nber.org/programs-projects/projects-and-centers/oregon-health-insurance-experiment?page=1&perPage=50

Rand Health Insurance Experiment: https://www.rand.org/pubs/research_briefs/RB9174.html

Pro-con debates mentioned in this book:

Medicare Advantage debate: we recommend reading this article as well as the four articles it references (linked to in the text).

- "The Debate on Overpayment in Medicare Advantage: Pulling It Together," *Health Affairs Forefront*. Published February 24, 2022. doi:10.1377/forefront.20220223.736815

Physician and Nurse Practitioner equivalence.

- For an opinion stating they are not equivalent, read Sandeep Jauhar's *New York Times* article from April 29, 2014, titled "Nurses Are Not Doctors."

- For an opinion supporting NP independent practice, read John Mandrola's *Medscape* article from January 22, 2020, titled "Independent Nurse Practitioners and Physician Assistants: A Doc's View."

People to follow on Twitter

Adrianna McIntyre @onceuponA

Bob Wachter @Bob_Wachter

Farzad Mostashari @Farzad_MD

Kirsten Bibbins-Domingo @KBibbinsDomingo

Avik Roy @Avik

Lisa Bari @lisabari

Michael L Barnett @ml_barnett

Peter Bach @peterbachmd

Elisabeth Rosenthal @RosenthalHealth

David Grabowski @DavidCGrabowski

Capybaras @capybaracountry

Index

Note: Page numbers followed by *f*, *t* denote figures and tables respectively.

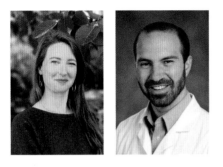

Elisabeth Askin and Nathan Moore are graduates of the MD program at the Washington University School of Medicine in St. Louis, Missouri. Elisabeth is a general internal medicine physician and associate clinical professor at the University of California-San Francisco, and Nathan is a general internal medicine physician with BJC Medical Group in St. Louis, medical director of the BJC Accountable Care Organization, and clinical assistant professor of medicine at Washington University in St. Louis. They both graduated from the University of Texas at Austin, met in medical school, and bonded over how much they missed breakfast tacos.

Elisabeth and Nathan are available for speaking engagements or for feedback and suggestions for future editions of this book. Please contact them via info@HealthCareHandbook.com.